A NEW
IBS
SOLUTION

BACTERIA—THE MISSING LINK IN
TREATING IRRITABLE BOWEL SYNDROME

MARK PIMENTEL, MD

HEALTH
P⊕INT
PRESS

COVER DESIGN: Jacqueline Michelus
EDITOR: Larry Trivieri
TYPESETTING AND BOOK DESIGN: Gary A. Rosenberg

Health Point Press
4335 Van Nuys Blvd
Sherman Oaks, CA 91403
818-788-2040

Library of Congress Cataloging-in-Publication Data

ISBN: 0-9774356-0-1

10   9   8   7   6   5

Contents

PART TWO
The IBS Treatment Plan:
Putting It All Together

To my loving wife, Ruchi,
and children, Maya and Luis (aka Weezi).
They are my life.

I would like to further dedicate this book
to my mother, Joanna,
and late father, Luis Pimentel,
who, by example, inspire a strong work ethic
and dedication to a task.

Acknowledgments

I have many people to thank for this book, but first and foremost, I need to thank the thousands of IBS patients I have encountered these past years. My research team is almost 10,000 strong. They, above all, were my instructors, my guides, and through their experience have changed IBS everywhere. What patients teach you cannot be learned in a book, and you must listen in order to hear and learn. If this book accomplishes only one thing I will be pleased: to empower people with IBS to realize that a pat on the head can no longer be an acceptable treatment for IBS.

I need to take the time to thank my mentors. Can you believe I am about to thank my chemistry teacher at Hammarskjold High School in Thunder Bay, Ontario, Mr. David Linklater? He loved chemistry with contagious enthusiasm. Another is Dr. Ken Van Ameyde. He taught me to listen for the medical clues from the patient and the art of bedside medicine (the traditional way). I need to include Dr. Charles Bernstein whose strong sense of academic drive reinforced my desire to pursue academic gastroenterology. I would particularly like to thank Dr. Henry C. Lin. He was instrumental in my training as a gut motility specialist and was a large part of the initial stages of this body of work. I would also like to thank Dr. Stephan R. Targan, Chief of the Division of Gastroenterology at Cedars-Sinai Medical Center. He has his eye trained on nurturing academic gastroenterologists and his legacy is still being written. I would particularly like to thank Dr.

Jeffery Conklin. There are rare people you meet in a lifetime who inspire an enthusiasm in what we do. He is a master clinician. We have much to learn from his generosity and friendship. I would also like to thank Dr. Edy Soffer for his contribution to the knowledge of small bowel physiology.

I also need to thank all those research personnel who worked so diligently to accomplish our wild notions (what a roller coaster for them). These include Dr. Evelyn Chow (the original), Sandy Park (my right hand), Yuthana Kong (my left hand), Christine Lee (our anchor), Brian Van den Burg, Fawzia Hegle (in it from the beginning), Robert Wade (aka "Bobby Wade, GIMT" and "the breath test guru"), Tess Constantino, RN (best motility nurse in the world), Vicky Lees-Kim, RN (also the best motility nurse in the world), and all the residents who have contributed to our research efforts. I am watching all of you! To thank Evelyn, Sandy, and Yuthana is simply not enough. They make the research happen and are the best one could hope to work with.

I would graciously like to express my gratitude to the amazing Larry Trivieri for his assistance in assembling this work. He has an ability to grasp and translate complex ideas. In addition, Cheri Singer from the Briefcase was instrumental in producing high-quality transcripts that eased the pain of editing. I would also like to thank copyeditor Lisa Kaspin and proofreader Carol Rosenberg for their editorial help.

I need to express my sincerest thanks to David Knight of BookTalk. He was the one catalyst for this book. "The time is right for a book to liberate patients with IBS based on your work." He understands the power of the written language to make a difference, and people with IBS need to benefit from this.

Although there are many other people to thank, I really need to express my most humble appreciation to Deanna and Hershel Levine from the Beatrice and Samuel A. Seaver Foundation in New York. New ideas and concepts are very difficult to get funded. The early intellectual stage of a bacterial concept in IBS was controversial. Agencies fund safe ideas—ideas with history. This foundation placed much trust in my efforts and has provided the bulk of the resources to generate the now cohesive body of scientific evidence that is presented in this book. In a similar fashion, Daniel Lundberg and many others from Salix Pharmaceuticals took significant risks in entering the IBS arena with our ideas. Who would have thought a ten-day course of antibiotics makes all the difference in IBS?

Lastly, I need to take the time to thank my wife, Ruchi, and children, Maya and Luis. The effort has required much time and their support makes it all possible. My wife is a brilliant research diabetologist/endocrinologist. Two academic physicians in one house make for interesting dinner conversation. She tells me that "hormones control the gut and that makes me your boss." Who can argue with that? *Me.* I say, "What would you do if I wasn't here?" I love my wife and kids. I would also like to thank my brother, Dan, as well as my father and mother, to whom this book is dedicated.

Introduction

Irritable bowel syndrome (IBS), characterized by abdominal pain, bloating, and altered bowel habits, is the most common chronic medical condition. Although there is some variation from study to study and country to country, up to 20 percent of a given population appears to be affected by this condition. In addition, unlike other chronic conditions such as heart disease, IBS commonly affects all ages. In fact, studies have shown that people with IBS have a lower quality of life than those with heart disease or other chronic medical conditions. Despite these facts, developments that may identify causes for IBS have happened only recently.

The progress to find a cause for IBS can hardly be called a race. The nature of the illness has interfered with that progress; most patients with IBS find it difficult to discuss their bowel problems with others and often suffer in silence. This may be due, in part, to the media's tendency to ridicule those with IBS or other digestive conditions such as lactose intolerance. All of these factors lead to social isolation and continued unwillingness to discuss the condition, further contributing to the patients' lower quality of life and the public's ignorance of IBS. One reason for our lack of knowledge about IBS is the lack of funding for research into its cause and treatment. Since IBS is not a fatal illness, it is not given priority for research funding. As a result, researchers who wish to unravel the IBS puzzle struggle to secure resources; fundraising takes up time those physicians would otherwise have for treating patients. Moreover, only a handful of researchers in the United States are working to identify a cause for IBS. The result is that most physicians continue to have a poor understanding about IBS. Often, when a disease is not clearly understood, the first inclination is to link the disease with the psychological condition of the patient. There are many historical examples of such thinking. In the 1970s, there was much discussion about the cardiac risk posed by having a "type A" personality. We now understand heart disease in a completely different way, and this reference is no longer part of the medical doctrine.

In another example, stress was thought to be the main cause of stomach ulcers until the discovery of the bacteria *Helicobacter pylori* as the most common culprit. With the inability of scientists to pinpoint the causes of IBS, people with IBS have fallen victim to psychological scrutiny and are often stigmatized as a result. In some cases, this stigma makes it difficult for IBS sufferers to obtain insurance policies, especially disability insurance.

To be fair, it is well known that a history of severe psychological trauma can lead to changes in bowel function. It is also understood that stress can influence the degree of symptoms in some IBS sufferers. However, it is now known that in most cases stress and psychological problems neither cause nor are associated with IBS. While this conclusion should be a victory for those with IBS, the stigma remains since the misconceptions run deep in the grassroots medical community.

Many factors have contributed to the declarations that IBS is more than psychological. For example, in non-university-based medical studies, the psychological profile of IBS patients is no different from the rest of the community. This discovery was paralleled by research contributing to the development of four new theories in IBS.

The discovery of altered pain perception in the gut was the first of four key findings. In the 1990s, studies demonstrated that IBS patients experienced gut pain at much lower thresholds than the general population. In other words, what would not be considered painful to the gut in normal subjects was perceived as painful in IBS patients. This led to innovative studies looking at pain processing in the gut and its transmission to the brain, or the "brain-gut axis." Brain imaging has since shown that IBS patients respond differently to pain; locations of the brain not otherwise activated by pain were being turned on in IBS. This work had several limitations; the techniques for measuring brain imaging required a high level of expertise and yielded inconsistent results among studies. Also, for patients, this concept has not easily translated into a better understanding of the causes and treatment of IBS.

One negative outcome of these findings was the initial marrying of these pain and brain findings to the older psychological theory of IBS. This union led investigators to consider antidepressant medications as a potential remedy. Since some antidepressants (especially tricyclic antidepressants such as amitriptyline) have also been shown to have numbing effects on the spine pain fibers (nerves), the fit was too tempting. While the ill effects of widespread antidepressant use had some in the scientific community concerned, studies showed that antidepressants could slow down bowel movements. Thus the concept that any antidepressant could work began to take hold. The ultimate consequence is that antidepressants have been a mainstay of IBS treatment. Shortly after the discovery of heightened sensation in the gut in IBS, others were taking a different scientific approach. One sentiment was that IBS was difficult to define because the disease was really a mixed group of conditions. The division of IBS into subcategories could in theory simplify its definition, making the causes more apparent. This approach led to the second theory of IBS, in which IBS is a group of disorders, with the dominant symptom defining each group. IBS with diarrhea as the main symptom would be labeled "diarrhea-predominant IBS"; and if constipation were the main feature, the label would read "constipation-predominant IBS." Efforts were also made to provide a clear definition of IBS. From this thinking was born what is now referred to as the Rome criteria.

Studies then emerged showing that for IBS patients suffering from constipation, intestinal movements were slower compared with normal controls. In contrast, in IBS patients suffering from diarrhea, the gut appeared to propel its contents too fast. Based on this, drug companies began to search for the chemicals produced by the gut that control its movement. A key chemical is serotonin, secreted by cells that line the gut wall. When food enters the area, serotonin is released, causing the gut to contract in a special fashion called "peristalsis." Peristalsis is a forward movement or spreading of gut contents such

as food down the gut. On a simplified level, if there is too much serotonin, there is too much movement; not enough and the gut is slower.
Some IBS studies demonstrated this connection between serotonin
levels and gut movement, which became the basis for a new class of
drugs that block (alosetron, cilansetron, granisetron) or augment
(tegaserod) the sites of action of serotonin.

The third theory of IBS stems from a pattern that investigators
began to recognize among patients with IBS who had suffered attacks
of acute diarrhea. Approximately 20 percent of IBS sufferers declare
that their bowel habits were perfectly normal until such an attack.
In most cases, the patients recall the incident as a clear case of food
poisoning, while in many other instances, the acute diarrhea began
on a trip abroad. Even after the acute episode of diarrhea subsides, the
bowel habits never return to normal. In light of this history, clinicians
aggressively investigated the stool for infective agents but found nothing, often years after the initial event. The recognition of this symptom
complex has led researchers from Europe and Canada to study food-
poisoning cases. Now, most researchers agree that a certain proportion
of food-poisoning cases will lead to perpetual IBS-like symptoms. This
idea of IBS being precipitated by an intestinal infection was termed
"post-infectious IBS."

The final, most recent theory defines IBS as a bacterial disease.
People with IBS inevitably complain of gas and bloating. While this
was once considered a major hallmark of IBS, the failure to understand this component led investigators in the 1980s to emphasize what
was more easily grasped; hence the focus on diarrhea and constipation. Still, even as most members of the scientific community were dis-
tracted by the emphasis on bowel function, others investigated the
bacterial component of IBS. In the 1990s, research showed that IBS
patients (over a given time) produced five times more gas than did
people without IBS. Since the only source of those gases was bacterial, the initial presumption was that IBS patients had excessive bacteria in the colon, where bacteria were expected to be. Subsequent
studies showed that IBS patients had excessive quantities of gas in the
small bowel; these data were the catalyst for studying small bowel
bacteria in IBS.

Normally, the small intestine contains a very small quantity of bacteria. In published studies, indirect measures of small bowel bacteria

suggest that 84 percent of IBS sufferers have excessive quantities of bacteria typically found in the colon.

Intuitively, higher bacterial levels in the small bowel, where absorption takes place, would ferment the nutrients from the food into gas. Further work in this area has determined that these bacteria could produce both constipation and diarrhea, depending on the types of bacteria that have moved into the small bowel. These results have led to studies showing that antibiotics can almost completely relieve IBS symptoms if successful in eliminating the intestinal bacteria. This is called the "bacterial overgrowth theory of IBS."

This book takes you through the evolution of thinking in IBS in a way that can be easily understood. The research is often complex even for those in the field; physicians and patients alike may get lost trying to understand the quagmire of opinions and research findings. In the desire for help, along with frustration with their physicians' limited understanding of how to treat IBS, many people have turned to alternative therapies such as probiotics. While some of these therapies have positive results, others are not as helpful and, in some rare cases, may be detrimental. These too will be discussed. While the initial chapters focus on how the theories of IBS diverge, the final chapters will show how the theories converge into a unifying hypothesis, and will give an indication of where IBS developments are heading in the future.

PART ONE

A New Understanding of Irritable Bowel Syndrome

CHAPTER 1

Breaking the Stigma:
IBS Is *Not* "All in Your Head"

I will never forget the day Margaret Anne (not her real name) first came to my office. "If you can't help me, I don't know what I will do," Margaret began, with a look that pleaded with me to help her. "I can't go on living like this!"

By *this*, Margaret was referring to her interminable struggle to find a way to properly address a health condition that had burdened her for many years, sapping her energy and severely affecting her ability to engage in the day-to-day activities that healthy people take for granted—simple things like grocery shopping or having lunch with friends—without the panicked feeling that she might have to cut things short because of an urgent need to go to the bathroom.

But these were not the only hurdles Margaret—sixty-five years old and clearly an intelligent woman—had to contend with. Like countless other patients, Margaret had repeatedly been told by many physicians over the years that nothing was physically wrong with her. Their unanimous diagnosis was that Margaret's gastrointestinal disorder was due to stress and depression, resulting in irritable bowel syndrome, or IBS. Margaret came to believe them, accepting their recommendation that she try antidepressants to control her emotions and possibly her bowel dysfunction as well.

While the medications left her feeling calmer, they did nothing to lessen her complaints. She still experienced altered bowel habits, abdominal pain, and the associated fears of eating—especially in public places—that are so common to people in Margaret's situation. Yet the more Margaret told her physicians that their prescriptions were not working, the more they told her the problems were "all in her head." Their response to the failing drug treatment was to increase the dose and, when that didn't work, to add more drugs.

By the time Margaret came to see me, she was taking three antidepressant medications, as well as two other prescription drugs to ease the constipation caused by the antidepressants. Her bowel situation had in fact worsened because of the side effects of the antidepressants. No wonder the poor woman told me she couldn't go on living like this.

To me, the saddest thing about Margaret's predicament was the fact that all her pain and uncertainty were unnecessary. Margaret's problems were not "all in her head," nor were they caused by stress or depression. Just like millions of Americans with similar symptoms, Margaret was a victim of the traditional medical approach to a poorly defined illness. The result is ongoing pain and discomfort, as well as the shame associated with the stigma of being diagnosed with a psychological disease.

A simple breath test for the presence of intestinal bacteria was conducted on Margaret. The test showed that her problems were due to an abnormally high concentration of bacteria in her small intestine (otherwise known as "small intestinal bacterial overgrowth"), which, as you shall learn, is being shown to be a possible cause of IBS.

Once the test results were in, I told Margaret, "I don't think your problem is psychological." As many others before and since, she looked at me with a mixture of hope and disbelief. How could I be so sure I could help her when so many doctors had not? I asked her to trust me, and then prescribed a course of antibiotics along with dietary recommendations (which you will also learn about later in this book). Margaret left my office with the promise that she would try my approach.

Two weeks later, Margaret came back to see me. The transformation she had undergone since her first visit was dramatic. Gone was the sad, burdened woman at her wit's end. In her place was an obviously healthy and vibrant woman with an entirely new lease on life. It wasn't that the therapy cured her depressive symptoms so much as it normalized her bowel function, validating her claim "the problem is in my gut." In her hand, she carried a brown bag, the contents of which she dumped on my desk. I looked down to see the bottles containing the five medications she had been placed on before our first visit.

"Thank you, doctor," she said, her face aglow with a beaming smile. "I no longer need these!" I administered another breath test, which confirmed that the antibiotics had done their job. Her bacterial overgrowth was a thing of the past and, with it, all of the unexplained bowel symptoms Margaret had suffered with for so many years.

Margaret's turnaround may seem amazing, especially to readers who suffer from IBS and struggle to find a solution to their problem, but most IBS cases are like Margaret's. More important, you can experience the same relief that Margaret did, once you read about the research seeking the cause of IBS and learn about treatments based on that research. But first, I want to explain why IBS is routinely and often inaccurately thought to be "all in a patient's head." From my perspective, it is this label and the stigma it places on people with IBS that lie at the heart of why so many millions of people continue to needlessly suffer in silence.

IBS: THE PSYCHOLOGICAL LABEL

Why is IBS so commonly thought to have psychological origins?

Until recently, most physicians have not clearly understood IBS, much less its cause. All that was known was that stress can alter bowel function and frequency; during times of acute stress, people often have diarrhea or experience nausea or other gastrointestinal disturbances. As a result, since the 1970s, IBS has routinely been thought by health professionals to result from stress and/or related psychological disturbances.

The medical community has a history of considering stress to be a possible factor in poorly understood conditions that are later deemed to have more practical causes. Perhaps the most famous example of this is the "type A personality," routinely accepted by doctors as a strongly associated factor in heart disease and other cardiovascular conditions.

While stresses related to the lifestyles of people with such a personality can contribute to heart disease (as well as to many other dis-

IBS at a Glance

IBS stands for *irritable bowel syndrome,* a functional disorder of the colon and intestines that is characterized by:

> ➤ Abdominal pain

> ➤ Diarrhea, constipation, or both

> ➤ Bloating

> ➤ Gas (flatulence)

> ➤ Urgency

Less well-known features include sleep disturbances, fatigue, fibromyalgia, belching, and occasionally nausea.

Some people suffering from IBS may be able to tolerate the symptoms enough to go about their daily life, but for many people, the pain and uncertainty of bowel function can be disabling enough to prevent them from working, traveling, and even socializing.

The incidence of IBS in the United States is quite high, ranging from 10 to 20 percent of the general population. Similar prevalence rates are seen in most other industrialized nations around the world. In the United States, IBS is the number-one disorder diagnosed by gastroenterologists (physicians who specialize in treating gastrointestinal disorders) and is the most common chronic medical condition.

While IBS is not considered serious because its symptoms are not life threatening, people with IBS often experience a poor quality of life that is worse than that experienced by sufferers of other chronic diseases, including cardiovascular illness.

The cause of IBS is often misdiagnosed because when the colon and intestines are examined (during tests such as colonoscopy), no signs of physical damage are visible. For this reason, IBS patients are frequently and unfairly told their condition is "all in their head" and are prescribed antidepressants with the expectation that these drugs will help their bowel habits along with their stress. Though many IBS patients *are* understandably anxious or depressed as a result of their condition, stress and other emotional problems are *not* the primary cause of IBS.

ease conditions), we now know how important other factors such as diet, exercise, cholesterol, blood pressure, homocysteine levels, and even chronic infection are to heart health. Given this new knowledge, physicians today would be making a big mistake if stress were the only factor they treated in their heart patients.

Until recently, another common health problem—peptic, or stomach, ulcer—was also thought to be linked primarily to stress and, to a lesser extent, the overuse of aspirin and nonsteroidal anti-inflammatory drugs (NSAIDs). For a physician to suggest otherwise was to risk rejection, ridicule, and even ostracism by the rest of the medical community. This is precisely what happened to the Australian doctors J. Robin Warren, a pathologist, and Barry Marshall, a gastroenterologist, about two decades ago when they first presented evidence that more than 90 percent of cases of peptic ulcer were caused by a bacterium in the gastrointestinal tract later known to be *Helicobacter pylori* (*H. pylori*).

Since then, not only have their findings been confirmed but antibacterial drugs are now the primary accepted form of treatment for chronic peptic ulcers, while stress is only addressed in the few cases in which it actually plays a role. In fact, the website of the Centers for Disease Control and Prevention states the following about ulcers: "While stress and diet can irritate an ulcer, they do not cause it. Ulcers are caused by the bacterium *H. pylori*, and can be cured with a one- or two-week course of antibiotics, even for people who have had ulcers for years." (Source: www.cdc.gov/ulcer/myth.htm)

As the evidence presented in this book will make clear, bacterial overgrowth is now being found in a growing number of IBS patients, and is beginning to be recognized as a potential cause. However, as happened with Warren's and Marshall's evidence that *H. pylori* was the primary cause of peptic ulcers, new research takes time to be validated and accepted by the general medical community and, consequently, patients on a widespread basis. Most physicians still equate IBS with stress and therefore prescribe a protocol similar to Margaret's antidepressant regimen, with equally poor results.

Besides the misunderstanding of the cause of IBS, there are even more complex reasons why IBS is thought to have psychological rather than physical causes. Research in IBS was burgeoning in the 1970s, at a time when endoscopy (direct visualization of the intestines with cameras) was in a renaissance. The excitement in endoscopy came with the introduction of flexible fiberoptic devices, cameras for looking into the gut. These devices allowed better-than-ever visualization of the intestines and consequently focused the field of gastroenterology on diseases you can see with the naked eye. This was a big shift from the study of gut physiology (function) as a basis for diagnosing patients. Since then, practice has become all about scoping, which is easy and profitable. Possible disease causes were only recognized if they could be visualized with an endoscope; patients with nothing "visibly" wrong were thought of as "difficult" because finding answers took effort and was not lucrative.

In addition, stress is known to alter bowel function and frequency; during times of acute stress, people can often have diarrhea or experience nausea or other gastrointestinal disturbances. The difference between such disturbances and IBS is that the former are usually acute or not long lasting, whereas IBS symptoms are perpetual even after the stress has passed. Even so, with the recognition of stress effects on gut function, along with the 1970s endoscopy renaissance, the stage was set for the subsequent two decades of research associating IBS with psychology and stress.

The following scenario, which many of my patients have lived through before they came to see me, illustrates this.

After enduring painful gastrointestinal symptoms for a number of months, a patient finally consented to see a doctor. The doctor performed a physical exam and found nothing wrong with her, then asked, "Does stress make your bowels worse?" "Yes," she replied. "When I am really stressed my symptoms are worse."

Hearing this, the doctor nodded his head knowingly, saying, "Your symptoms are due to IBS because it is stress-related. I'm going to write you a prescription for the anxiety you're feeling."

"But, doctor," the patient said, "I'm having symptoms even when I'm not stressed . . . even when I'm on holiday or just relaxing around the house."

The woman knows that stress isn't causing her symptoms, only aggravating them, but the doctor focuses on stress when choosing the treatment. The woman will start taking the pills prescribed (such as antianxiety drugs or antidepressants), but her symptoms won't abate. Frustration then mounts, creating a vicious and unnecessary cycle of further stress that only makes things worse while the cause of her condition remains undefined.

Another point that must be made is that the patients, regardless of the type of bowel condition, only experience a few types of symptoms (pain, diarrhea, or constipation). Thus, not only is it important to rule out stress as the cause of the patient's presenting symptoms, it is also necessary to rule out other conditions that can appear similar to IBS, such as colitis, Crohn's disease, gastroesophageal reflux disease (GERD), infection, inflammatory conditions of the stomach, and even colon cancer.

In defense of this work, severe psychological stress, such as sexual or physical abuse, are traumatic events, and associations drawn between these traumatic events and bowel dysfunction are real. If nothing else, the research helped physicians identify those with serious issues that privately haunted many patients. In most cases, this was trauma that needed healing and appropriate management, and this effort should never be underappreciated. At the same time, many of these studies were conducted at centers of excellence for integrating gastroenterology and psychiatry, leading to selection for a population with previous psychological trauma. Recent evidence now suggests that in the general community of IBS, psychological disorders are no different between people suffering with IBS and those who are not.

SUFFERING IN SILENCE

There is one particular stress that comes with IBS: the stigma attached to the disease, which forces patients to suffer in silence. I am speaking about the reticence of people with IBS to speak about it. Let's face it. Talking about our bowel habits under any circumstance is hardly a comfortable thing to do, and is hardly a topic of conversation in polite society. For most people, doing so would leave them embarrassed, even shamed. So it's no wonder that people who have IBS are reluctant to tell others, even their own physician in some cases. And, when they do speak to their doctors about it, once they are reassured that IBS isn't fatal, all too often they resign themselves to the belief that they "just have to live with it," and then may not discuss their condition any further.

The Fallacy and Dangers of Prescribing Antidepressants for IBS

While I am certainly not opposed to the judicious use of antidepressant medications under appropriate circumstances, I believe that in many cases such drugs are being prescribed when they are, in fact, unnecessary. This is particularly true with regard to IBS.

The conditions for which antidepressants may prove helpful—severe and chronic anxiety and depression—are not the cause of IBS. It's important to note that not all IBS patients suffer from pronounced anxiety or depression. In fact, surveys show that the incidence of anxiety and depression are no greater among IBS patients than among the general population. Therefore, from my perspective, it usually does not help to prescribe antidepressants for IBS, since such drugs are incapable of addressing what causes IBS—such as the unchecked overgrowth of bacteria in the gastrointestinal tract. Nevertheless, initial studies of antidepressants showed some promise. Although much time was spent suggesting that IBS is part of a psychological disorder and this is the basis for antidepressant therapy, specific antidepressant drugs do have other properties that make them an understandable choice to treat IBS. Specifically, amitriptyline (a tricyclic antidepressant) not only helps with anxiety and depression, but also has been shown to have properties that help in reducing pain. Furthermore, a side effect of amitriptyline is constipation, which can help ease diarrhea-predominant IBS. These added benefits were also fuel for the argument that antidepressants may be helpful.

A major problem with early studies (especially of antidepressants) in IBS was the outcome measures used. One of the few validated scoring systems for IBS studies was the IBS-QOL (IBS Quality of Life Score). The problem with this and other early scoring systems is that most of the questions are related to psychology. To put it simply, using a psychology based scoring system in IBS as the outcome measure in a study using an antidepressant suggests that the psychological results should be connected with the IBS symptoms.

To use an analogy, if a patient with IBS was given a blood pressure medication and, after using it, his blood pressure levels improved, whether or not his IBS symptoms improved, would it make sense to say that blood pressure medications are a solution for IBS because the pressure dropped? Of course not. This is evident from a recent study in which subjects received an antidepressant for IBS. This time, the psychology scores were separated from the bowel complaint scores. The antidepressants improved psychological scores but did little for the bowel habits. In other words, antidepressants improved the depressive symptoms (which we already knew) in IBS patients (it does this for all patients) but did not improve IBS. Moreover, in a recent study by a respected investigator, Douglas Drossman, MD, designed to specifically show once and for all that tricyclic antidepressants work for IBS, the results were mostly negative.

Besides antidepressants' limited effectiveness in IBS, there is another reason for concern about the use of antidepressants to treat people with IBS. Such drugs can cause serious side effects and can also prove to be addictive over time, making it difficult for patients to stop using them. According to Joseph Glenmullen, PhD, an expert in this area, side effects of antidepressant medications can include uncontrollable facial and body tics, dizziness, hallucinations, nausea, sexual dysfunction, and possible neurological damage and permanent structural change to the brain, due to how these drugs affect brain chemistry. In some cases, the drugs can even lead to suicide and antisocial, even homicidal, behavior. All of these factors are why I am so reluctant to prescribe them for my IBS patients.

Compounding the problem is the social stigma attached to bowel dysfunction in general and IBS in particular. Comedians poke fun at it, and even friends and family members may joke about it. Just a few weeks ago, I happened to watch a popular sitcom. In the episode, the characters were teasing someone about having IBS. Would your friends tease you in the same way if they knew you had IBS? We wouldn't expect to see a television comedy teasing a man with diabetes or kidney disease, so why should it be acceptable to make fun of people with IBS? But it still happens, leading to more reluctance to discuss this problem.

Another factor that adds to the public silence about IBS has to do with the association of IBS with psychological disorders. On first experience, many patients, when they find the courage to admit they are experiencing bowel dysfunction, are then turned off when their physicians subject them to the extensive psychological history as part of the accepted medical protocol for treating IBS. Many of these patients are concerned about where such questioning is leading and, rather than having their answers entered into their medical records, choose to curtail their appointment and continue to suffer in silence. For the alternative is to be tagged as a patient with mental health issues: those issues become part of their medical records for all time.

An even more ominous scenario is how health-insurance coverage can be affected. Over the years, I have been told by a number of patients that listing IBS as one of their health conditions was likely to compromise their health coverage. Health-insurance providers consider IBS patients to be high users, more likely to go on disability than patients with other chronic health conditions. As a result, many people find that admitting they have IBS can have serious consequences when it comes to paying for their health care or obtaining disability insurance.

CONCLUSION

For all of the reasons mentioned in this chapter, public awareness of IBS and the serious health concerns associated with it remain low, despite the high incidence of IBS in our country and other industrialized nations. Breaking the silence and stigma that surrounds IBS and, far more important, empowering the millions of people who suffer from it with a proven method for treating it are the reasons I wrote this book. As you read through the remaining chapters, you will begin to see how new theories (especially the concept of bacterial overgrowth) will unfold. In Chapter 2, we will take a look at IBS subgroups to educate you on terminology used by physicians.

CHAPTER 2

Too Fast or Too Slow:

Understanding Your IBS Symptoms

"**M**y friend was given a diagnosis of IBS, but she has diarrhea three times a day. Meanwhile, I'm constipated most of the time. My doctor said I have IBS too. Since our symptoms are so different, how can we both have IBS?"

Comments like the one above are quite common. The problem, as mentioned in Chapter 1, is that the cause of IBS is unknown. Furthermore, there is no blood test to diagnose it. In the absence of such tests, physicians tend to think of IBS as a "diagnosis of exclusion." A diagnosis of exclusion in medicine means that a patient has been examined (usually with some testing being done) and though the causes of the symptoms are not readily apparent, the condition is still given a label. When the symptoms involve changes in bowel function with no identifiable cause, that label is usually IBS. Since the gut symptoms generally only include constipation or diarrhea, these too become labels for IBS, that is, predominantly constipation or predominantly diarrhea. The categorization is, in fact, more complicated than that.

Before discussing the categorization in detail, the most important step in diagnosing IBS is being able to say for certain that a patient does not have something else. Certain factors determine the scrutiny needed. In one of the more serious cases, people older than age fifty with a change in bowel function warrant more intense investigation mostly due to an increased risk of colon cancer in this age category. For such patients, colonoscopy (camera visualization of the colon) would then be needed. Other considerations include Crohn's disease and celiac disease in situations where diarrhea is the main feature. The possibility that there is a more ominous condition can at times weigh heavily on people. Patients often ask questions such as "Are you sure there isn't something else wrong besides IBS?" Most clinicians have examples of patients initially labeled by another physician with IBS; the patients are later found to have pancreatic cancer or Crohn's disease. All of the anxiety rests on the fact that there is no definitive test for IBS. As such, some clinicians even look at the term "IBS" as a catchall acronym with little meaning, a label that amounts to nothing.

There is another problem with the use of diagnosis of exclusion as a determinant of IBS: if you do find what looks like a cause, then it cannot be IBS. For example, as we began to publish data (discussed later in more detail) showing that a large proportion of IBS patients appear to have too much bacteria in the small intestine (bacterial overgrowth), one criticism was "If you find bacterial overgrowth in a patient, then the patient can't have IBS." When one of my research papers was published, the journal received a letter from a scientist who stated that he couldn't fathom how I could have found an association between IBS and bacterial overgrowth, because if bacterial overgrowth is present then the patients' symptoms can't be due to IBS. This person is not alone in making this assumption. In other words, if out of one hundred possible IBS patients, eighty have bacterial overgrowth, now you have only twenty patients with true IBS. This way of thinking about IBS would never allow researchers to identify a cause.

Amidst all this confusion about defining IBS, and now with the association with bacterial overgrowth, I have had numerous patients ask me, "What should I call my condition? Do I have IBS or am I just suffering from bacterial overgrowth?"

I explain that it doesn't really matter what the label is. What matters is that identification of a treatable condition associated with IBS provides a way to treat their condition and give them the lasting relief they desire.

For those with a longer history of IBS, there is more confusion since every decade or so it seems to be renamed. In the 1960s and 1970s, it was called "non-specific colitis;" in the 1970s and 1980s, it became known as "spastic colon." Today, it's primarily known as IBS.

More recently, some researchers are leaning toward renaming it yet again, this time to functional bowel disease, IBS type.

An even more intriguing spin on IBS was the labeling of subgroups, which confuses patients even more. These labels include diarrhea- or constipation-predominant IBS. Although I stated above that IBS is a "diagnosis of exclusion," there needs to be criteria for patients to meet before the IBS label is applied. The most recent IBS criteria are called the "Rome criteria," which provide for subcategorization of IBS. The Rome criteria are so named because a group of gastrointestinal scientists/IBS experts developed the symptoms list at their first meeting in Rome, Italy. However, these scientists developed the criteria for research purposes only; therefore, these criteria have never been properly validated as a method of diagnosing IBS in a doctor's office. In order to standardize patient enrollment across the world, especially for drug studies, clinical criteria were still needed. Still, from the Rome criteria, the subcategorization of IBS into diarrhea-predominant and constipation-predominant types evolved.

IBS patients need to know what the Rome criteria are, should their physicians use it as a diagnostic method. Basically, the Rome criteria are used for convenience purposes, to label patients, but the criteria don't really address their symptoms and what might be causing them.

There were two reasons to subcategorize IBS. The first was because it was considered hard to explain the research findings occurring in the 1980s and 1990s without dividing IBS into those two categories. It was thought that IBS patients were a mixed population, because patients' complaints were mixed (some had more diarrhea-related symptoms; some had more constipation). So rather than trying to explain IBS as a whole, subcategorizing it would help researchers find a cause more easily. This approach is very similar to taking square pegs that don't fit into round holes. Instead of investigating more thoroughly where the pegs (the research findings) properly belonged, we simply chose to make the round holes (the clinical findings) square, to make everything already known fit together.

The second reason that IBS was divided into the categories of diarrhea- and constipation-predominant types had to do with treatment options. We had medication that made people have constipation, and this would be good if someone had diarrhea. Likewise, we knew how to induce loosened stools in people with constipation. For constipa-

The Rome Criteria

The Rome criteria are divided into two sections:

1. Patients must have three months of abdominal pain that

   a) May be relieved by having a bowel movement;

   b) Is associated with altered stool frequency; or,

   c) Is associated with altered stool form or consistency.

2. Patients must have have two or more of the following symptoms for at least 25 percent of the time:

   a) A change in stool frequency of either diarrhea (more than three bowel movements a day) or constipation (fewer than three bowel movements a week);

   b) A difference in stool form (harder or looser);

   c) Passage of mucus during defecation;

   d) Bloating or abdominal distension;

   e) Altered passage of stool (feeling that not all the stool has come out after bowel movements, straining, urgency to pass bowel movements).

tion, physicians can suggest fiber, laxatives, and so forth. If diarrhea is the predominant symptom, then antidiarrhea medications such as Imodium can be prescribed. In both cases, this approach to drug therapy fails because it does not address IBS as a whole. IBS is not diarrhea alone or constipation alone but rather a constellation of symptoms including pain, bloating, and urgency.

Based on a published review of the scientific literature that I conducted, there has only been one published paper that validates the Rome criteria in terms of its ability to diagnose IBS, and it did not appear until years after the criteria were established. By contrast, the previous criteria used—the Manning criteria, established in 1978—were validated by multiple published papers, but this does not solve the problem because of the previously discussed limitations. Currently, most physicians rely upon the Rome 2 criteria, which were created by the same scientists following a second visit to Rome; so far there are no published papers validating the Rome 2 criteria as a valid diagnostic method for determining IBS at all.

Returning to the role that bacterial overgrowth plays in IBS, patients need to understand that the Rome criteria do not consider bacterial involvement. So, unless doctors are already familiar with the research I am sharing in this book, they may not even consider bacterial overgrowth as a possible cause for their patients' symptoms and therefore may not treat it. As you will discover in later chapters, there are various types of symptoms resulting from the bacterial overgrowth that causes IBS (at least in the majority of cases). For example, methane gas emitted from bacteria in the gastrointestinal tract appears to interfere with the body's elimination process, slowing down the transit time of waste material to cause constipation. Other people may experience diarrhea as a result of how the bacterial overgrowth affects them. Based on our research, my colleagues and I have been able to categorize the various bacteria involved into subtypes with corresponding symptoms. This reunifies IBS under one causative umbrella with different symptoms resulting from different physiologic consequences of one cause, and not from different causes. That will be explained later. For now, I want to emphasize once again that it is not the symptoms of IBS that matter most, but what is causing them. Regardless of whether your symptoms are diarrhea or constipation, don't be confused or upset. Rather, read on to learn how new findings suggest a potential cause and treatment of IBS.

In the 1980s, studies showed that in cases of diarrhea-predominant IBS, the gut is moving too fast, whereas in constipation-predominant IBS, it is moving too slow. This was the first hint that there was a gut problem in IBS. Work continued in this area while much of the public attention was focused on psychological aspects of IBS.

Various pharmaceutical companies succeeded in funding investigations of gut-movement abnormalities in IBS and for practical purposes began the conversion from psychology and the "garbage bag" diagnosis of IBS to promoting the concept that IBS is a "real" condition with measurable movement abnormalities.

THE SEROTONIN CONNECTION

The more that researchers examined the issue of motility as it related to diarrhea-predominant and constipation-predominant IBS, the more they focused their attention on serotonin, a chemical that controls peristalsis—the speed at which waste products and other things move through the gastrointestinal tract. This is understandable, since 95 percent of the body's serotonin is found in the gastrointestinal tract, with the remaining 5 percent located in the brain. Moreover, the more serotonin there is, the more aggressively things move through the gastrointestinal tract, while the less serotonin there is, the less aggressive is the rate of peristalsis.

There are a number of other chemical compounds that also affect peristalsis and contribute to hypersensitivity in the gastrointestinal tract, yet researchers initially focused on serotonin, which eventually led to a number of drugs to mediate gastrointestinal serotonin levels. The first of these was the drug alosetron, developed by Glaxo Wellcome (now GlaxoSmithKline), and marketed under the name Lotronex. This was the first serotonin drug specifically for IBS that received approval by the Food and Drug Administration (FDA) as a treatment for IBS. The intended purpose of alosetron was to slow down the fast transit time in diarrhea-predominant cases of IBS.

Alosetron accomplished this by acting as a complete blocker of serotonin receptor sites along the walls of the gastrointestinal tract, which is where serotonin causes the chain of events that control gut movements.

Alosetron was not without problems. For one thing, it worked not by slowing down gut movement but by shutting off much of the movement altogether. This is not something that you want to have happen, since movement must be present in order for the intestines to properly eliminate wastes and perform other important digestive functions. Shutting down gut movement led to severe constipation in up to 30 percent of IBS patients receiving the drug.

But the far more serious side effect of alosetron was that it caused ischemic colitis. This was something that was known prior to the drug's initial labeling, yet at the time, the reported 1 percent incidence of this complication was considered low. Ischemic colitis is a serious medical issue characterized by insufficient blood flow to the colon, which can cause bleeding into the gut, breakdown of the colon, and even death. Soon after FDA approval, severe constipation and numerous cases of ischemic colitis began to be reported, although more recent data suggest that ischemic colitis was less common than previously estimated due to earlier misdiagnosis. Still, in some cases, the side effects were severe enough that colon removal was needed, and even severe enough that patients died. Eventually, alosetron was removed from the market. Today, the drug is available in a limited fashion and is very difficult to obtain.

Currently, other drugs are being considered by the FDA as serotonin 3 receptor blockers similar to alosetron. One of them—cilansetron—is in clinical trials, and cases of ischemic colitis have already been noted. Solvay recently received a "non-approvable" letter from the FDA regarding this drug. What this means is that currently there is no serotonin-based class of drugs that has been shown to be safe for managing the symptoms of diarrhea-predominant IBS.

For constipation-predominant IBS, however, the drug tegaserod, marketed under the brand name Zelnorm, can be beneficial. Tegaserod's effects are the opposite of alosetron; it is not known to slow blood flow to the colon and so does not cause ischemic colitis. It is designed to act similarly to serotonin; in addition, it is not overly stimulating. It is just strong enough to get the job done, but not strong enough to cause dangerous side effects. In addition, it can be monitored and safely increased or decreased, depending on the needs of the individual. In addition, it has demonstrated significant effectiveness in managing constipation-predominant IBS.

However, there is some confusion about tegaserod because the clinical trials primarily involved female patients. In the two pivotal studies in the United States that demonstrated tegaserod's efficacy, one study completely involved women, and the other was composed almost entirely of women. As a result, I've had male patients call me from their local pharmacy, asking, "Do you know that this drug is only approved for women?"

At this point the difference between men and women in IBS needs to be discussed, because drug therapy appears more effective in women. The tegaserod studies involved primarily women for two reasons. First, women with IBS tend to respond better to drug therapy than men. Secondly, epidemiologic studies suggest that more women than men suffer from IBS. On the other hand, women tend to be far more likely to see a doctor and report their symptoms, compared with men, who all too often will keep their symptoms to themselves and are more reticent to seek medical advice.

Women, in general, have a more rigorous and earlier health-maintenance strategy (breast examination, Pap smears) than men and are thus more likely to see their doctors on a regular basis. Health maintenance in women often begins in their thirties, while most men don't start having regular prostate exams and colonoscopies until they are in their fifties.

One difference between women and men is harder to explain. Women are far more likely to experience chronic constipation than men. In my practice, I never see in men the same kind of constipation that I see in women. An extreme form of constipation is called "colonic inertia," in which patients have a bowel movement as infrequently as once a month. It's very rare for men to suffer from constipation to the same degree.

Although these gender differences are important in IBS, Novartis included men in their most recent FDA-approved indication for constipation. This is based on new data and clinical experience where it appears clear that the response to tegaserod is not gender dependent and can be used quite successfully in both groups.

METOCLOPRAMIDE (REGLAN): PROCEED WITH CAUTION

The abovementioned drugs make up part of the class of drugs that either block or stimulate serotonin receptors. Another drug that is sometimes used to promote movement of the gut is metoclopramide (Reglan). Its actions primarily affect the upper part of the gastrointestinal tract, not necessarily the colon itself. Metoclopramide is prescribed for a variety of conditions, including IBS, especially of the constipation-predominant variety. For some time now, I have not prescribed metoclopramide due to the side effects of the drug. Although the most common side effect is drowsiness or sedation, much more serious reactions occur such as extrapyramidal side effects, which include involuntary twitching of the muscles.

Even more ominously, patients may develop tardive dyskinesia, a condition characterized by permanent facial contortion. People who experience tardive dyskinesia after taking metoclopramide will continue to have it to some degree even after they discontinue using the drug.

Despite such side effects, a number of physicians and hospital staff members still prescribe metoclopramide because it is generic and therefore inexpensive. Because of its affordability alone, many people—physicians and patients alike—resist cautions against its use.

PLACEBO EFFECT?

Another concept that patients may hear about in IBS, and in general, is the placebo effect. A placebo is a pill that does not contain any active ingredients, for example a sugar pill. In the placebo effect, a certain percentage of patients—some estimates are as high as 30 percent—report improvement in their conditions while taking placebo because of their eagerness to feel better. This improvement also happens in combination with simple doctor contact through a study protocol.

In the case of IBS, the placebo effect has helped foster the belief that the symptoms are entirely psychological. Though it is true that some patients do seem to improve after receiving a placebo, this is by no means proof that their condition was "all in their head." Rather, it probably means that, as a result of being in the study, they pay more and better attention to their symptoms, and focus on the good rather than the bad, leading to their reports of improvement. In addition, because bowel symptoms fluctuate so much in IBS with or without treatment, it becomes easy for patients to convince themselves that they are getting better.

But there's another reason for the placebo effect in IBS patients that is due to what is known as "a soft versus a hard end point." Let's suppose that a drug company wants to determine the effectiveness of its blood-pressure medication. One way the company could do this would be to create a study in which patients with high blood pressure are given an electronic monitoring device to wear in the form of a bracelet. The electronic bracelet would be connected to a computer. During the clinical trial, subjects would be divided into two groups—those who receive the actual blood pressure medication, and those who receive a placebo drug. Throughout the trial period, the electronic bracelet would continue to monitor each patient's blood pressure levels and the patients would have no control over the reading the computer would score during that time. Such a test completely eliminates the patients' subjective feelings and therefore safeguards against the placebo effect. Either the blood pressure medication is effective or it is not. Either way, it is the electronic monitoring device that is reporting that answer, not the patients. This is what is known as "a hard end point outcome."

In determining the effectiveness of IBS treatments, however, such objective evaluations are missing. Instead, patients fill out questionnaires in which they report whether or not they are feeling better. Relying on questionnaires makes for a subjective, qualitative outcome report, not an objective, quantitative report like the one in the example above. Patients are asked questions such as: Is your abdominal pain better? If so, by what percentage has it improved? The answer to this will depend on many factors such as symptoms that day or general mood. Yet physicians rely on such questionnaires to let them know whether or not their IBS patients are getting better because currently we lack a quantitative tool for measuring their actual—not subjective—improvement. This is what is known as "a soft end point outcome."

Because of this fact, it is easy to dismiss results of clinical trials such as those in which subjects with constipation-predominant IBS were given tegaserod. Those studies found that tegaserod resulted in a 10 to 20 percent improvement over the placebo, which is statistically very significant. Yet critics still maintain that tegaserod really doesn't work any better than a placebo because it "only" increased improvement rates by 10 to 20 percent. The same degree of improvement is often achieved by drugs commonly used to treat Crohn's disease and all types of colitis—diseases of the gastrointestinal tract that modern medicine knows are non-psychological in nature. Or, if they do realize this, critics don't object to it in the same way because physicians can objectively measure improvements in patients with Crohn's disease or colitis by determining whether or not physical symptoms like bleeding and ulcers are improving, in addition to reviewing their responses on questionnaires.

The fact is that the effectiveness of drugs used to treat many disease conditions is on par with that of IBS drugs such as tegaserod in terms of the separation between placebo and the drugs' effectiveness, yet we don't criticize the other drugs in the same way. Again, this points to the stigma of IBS's being a psychological condition and the placebo effect's being a psychological phenomenon.

Overall, 45 to 60 percent of constipation-predominant IBS patients who use tegaserod will experience some degree of improvement of their symptoms, depending upon the patient and the severity of the symptoms. However, since IBS is not caused by serotonin excess or deficiency, neither tegaserod nor any of the other drugs discussed in this chapter that are used to regulate serotonin levels can be expected to be completely effective. For a truly effective solution, we need to look elsewhere.

ON THE RIGHT TRACK

While none of the drugs discussed in this chapter provide an optimum solution for IBS, they nonetheless represent an important shift away from the label of IBS as a psychological disorder.

The research into the development of these drugs has opened the door for physicians and researchers to begin considering IBS as a physiological condition with specific physical symptoms that have nothing to do with a patient's mental or emotional state (aside from the fact that anxiety and emotional stress can exacerbate the physical symptoms).

The fact that there now is interest on the part of pharmaceutical companies to continue to explore the physiological causes and symptoms of IBS represents an important change in medicine's approach to treating the disease. In addition, because of their interest in fully understanding IBS, they are also allocating significant amounts of their research budgets for this purpose. Their commitment to "getting to the bottom" of the IBS puzzle will have a dramatic impact on our understanding of the disease.

Another benefit of this shift on the part of the pharmaceutical companies is that IBS patients are being humanized in current advertisements for drugs such as tegaserod. Today, we are increasingly seeing ads on television and in magazines that feature real people who are willing to admit that they suffer from IBS. The positive impact and hope that these ads provide IBS sufferers should not be overlooked. These ads go a long way toward once and for all breaking the stigma that for so long has been such a burden for people with IBS.

CONCLUSION

Because of the ongoing research, I think we can expect to see another generation of drugs specifically targeted at treating IBS. In the meantime, although none of the current drugs discussed in this chapter provide a full and complete solution for IBS, they can at least provide a degree of symptom relief for some patients. This is particularly true of tegaserod. For real, lasting solutions, we need a more comprehensive approach to the problem. I will address this solution in Part Two.

CHAPTER 3

Big Brain, Little Brain:
The Gut's Nerve Network

A lthough, as we saw in Chapter 1, IBS is most definitely *not* a condition that is "all in a patient's head," it's important to recognize the roles that both the brain and the gut play in IBS. Research conducted since the 1980s suggests that both the brain and the gut respond differently in people with IBS than they do in people who do not have IBS.

In 1980, researcher William Whitehead published the results of a study he conducted showing that when a balloon was inflated in the rectum, IBS patients experienced pain at a less inflated level than non-IBS patients. Whitehead's research suggested that in IBS patients, the gut experienced pain at a level different from normal, and that it did not require as great a stimulus for the pain to be triggered. Put another way, Whitehead's research showed that IBS patients felt more pain in the gut than non-IBS patients did. His study initiated the concept of gut hyperalgesia's (heightened pain sensitivity) association with IBS.

Based on Whitehead's findings, physicians and researchers began to consider whether the brains of IBS patients were processing pain differently than normal. This question led to further research using brain imaging, some of it conducted by Whitehead and his colleagues, with additional research conducted by researchers at the University of California, Los Angeles (UCLA). The UCLA researchers employed PET brain scans, which revealed that certain areas of the brains of IBS patients were more active during painful stimulation of the rectum when compared with the control group. The PET scans suggested that different pathways of activation in the brain occurred in IBS patients compared with healthy people. This clearly suggested a link between the brain and IBS, but researchers remained stymied, because they could not pinpoint what the problem was or where in the brain it was occurring.

Adding to the difficulty of finding the answer was that many of the IBS patients in these studies were using medications such as anti-depressants, which had been prescribed because their physicians thought IBS was a symptom of psychological issues. Because such drug usage was so common among the IBS test groups, it was difficult to tell whether the altered pathways of activation in the brain were being caused by IBS or by the medications.

Adding to the dilemma was research published in the medical journal *Gastroneurology* that involved a patient in one of the brain-imaging studies. In the published study, the author stated that the patient was narcotic dependent, meaning she was dependent on various narcotic medications. She complained of symptoms that were considered to be those of IBS, and the brain imaging showed altered pathways of activation in her brain. But when this woman was then given psychotherapy and weaned off the narcotic medications, her gut symptoms improved and there was a corresponding normalization in brain activity, as shown by subsequent brain imaging. The fact that this woman was included in this particular IBS study is remarkable to me, because I suspect that perhaps she didn't have IBS to begin with. Rather, her bowel symptoms were probably due to her heavy use of narcotics.

Unfortunately, many of the patients in these studies suffered from similar psychological issues and were also taking medications that can significantly alter healthy bowel function. As a result, from my perspective, the study results were less than clear. Given the type of patients involved, it's very difficult to say for certain what the brain-imaging studies actually meant or how the data should have been interpreted. Additionally, no one can say for sure how the patients' medications influenced the studies' findings. Despite these concerns, brain-imaging studies have played a dominant part in all subsequent medical symposia and conferences devoted to understanding IBS, and the role of "brain-gut axis" (the term given to the link between the brain and the gut) has remained a major topic of discussion.

How could gastroenterologists who treat IBS use this research? The findings were simply observations, not data that could be used to target the cause of IBS and therefore to develop an appropriate treatment regimen. Moreover, an unfortunate consequence of the focus on brain-imaging studies and the brain-gut axis was that it further reinforced the belief that IBS was "all in the patient's head," and therefore best treated with antidepressants and other medications used to treat psychological or central nervous system conditions. After all, many physicians reasoned, if IBS involves the brain, it supports a psychological nature to IBS. Actually, this isn't the case. The brain does play a role in IBS, but it is a role that is *physiological,* not *psychological.*

Among the research that makes this clear is that of Michael Gershon, PhD. In the late 1980s and early 1990s, instead of focusing on the brain or the gut directly, Gershon conducted research on the nerves that intervene between them. More specifically, on the nerves that communicate from the gut to the brain and central nervous system. As a result of this research, we now understand the connection between serotonin and the speed of movement through the gut. This research later led to the development of drugs that stimulated serotonin receptors to relieve constipation (tegaserod) or blocked serotonin receptors to relieve diarrhea (alosetron). Through his research, Gershon further showed that serotonin can influence the rate at which the food by-products pass through the gastrointestinal tract. As we discussed in Chapter 2, too much serotonin can cause diarrhea whereas too little serotonin can result in constipation. Regulating serotonin levels through various medications has become a popular way for physicians to try to help their IBS patients. However, I am unaware of any published studies that indicate that disruptions in serotonin levels are a primary factor in IBS.

Even so, one of the interesting aspects of the research by Gershon is how it confirms that the gut, or gastrointestinal tract, has a nerve network that, while integrated with the brain, is also highly independent of it. In fact, research suggests that the gastrointestinal tract actually contains more nerve tissue than the brain does. Philosophically, this makes sense, because the gastrointestinal tract is the most evolved organ system in the body, since it is also the oldest organ system found in nature. Worms, for example, have a highly developed gastrointestinal tract, whereas they lack kidneys and brains, having a rudimentary neural network. Every type of animal has a gastrointestinal tract. Overall, the brain is the newest system of the body, especially its frontal lobes that control higher mental functioning such as speech, language, and reasoning. By comparison, the gastrointestinal tract is the oldest and most evolved, as well as possibly the most complex, organ system; it has its own extensive nerve network, which can function independently. In fact, if all nerve connections to the brain were removed, the gastrointestinal tract would continue to function on its own.

An example of this is vagotomy, a medical procedure that involves the administration of pharmaceutical drugs to prevent function of the vagus nerve, which helps to control motor and sensory function. Even when the vagus nerve is deactivated by this procedure, the gastrointestinal tract continues to function independently.

In normal human function, because the gut's neural network is integrated with that of the brain, the networks communicate with each other. While there is no question that the brain contributes to gastrointestinal tract function, the gut is also able to work independently. For this reason, Gershon has labeled the brain and the gut "big brain" and "little brain," respectively. Some scientists, however, argue that it might be more proper to designate the gut as the "big brain," because of how old it is, in terms of evolution, and how capable it is of independent function.

Building upon the research of Gershon and other researchers, over the last five years, Yvette Tache, PhD of UCLA has significantly contributed to our understanding of cortisol-releasing factor (CRF), a hormone that is produced in the brain in response to stress. Whenever we experience stressful events, or continue to be stressed over unresolved past events, the brain produces CRF, which in turn produces an increase in adrenaline. The increased adrenaline levels provide us with the extra energy we need to deal with the stress. Tache's research shows that when CRF is produced, it triggers three physiological effects within the gastrointestinal tract. First, colon function speeds up, meaning that the colon will eliminate stool more frequently. Second, stomach function slows down so that the stomach doesn't empty its contents as often. The third effect caused by elevated CRF is that the small bowel starts to have fewer cleansing waves, which could favor bacterial overgrowth.

Based on my own experience in treating IBS, I do not think that stress and its resulting increase in CRF levels cause IBS, but I do think that stress can modify IBS symptoms through the mechanism of CRF. I also believe that other factors are involved during times of stress that can also exacerbate IBS symptoms; more research is required before these factors can be fully understood. But to say that stress is causing IBS is not accurate, as the vast majority of IBS patients can testify. My IBS patients, for example, when I first consult with them, all point out that their IBS symptoms remain present regardless of whether they are stressed out or completely relaxed. So, though I do believe that stress can make IBS symptoms worse at times through CRF and other factors, it does not cause IBS.

I would estimate that while most Americans are stressed in some way, not all of them are suffering from IBS, even though stress can affect their gut function. This is an important point. In addition, we need to recognize that stress is often an aspect of activities we enjoy, including our jobs. Therefore, my role as a physician is not to tell my patients—with IBS or otherwise—to get a less stressful job than they currently have, because they may enjoy what they do for a living. (Managing stress effectively and appropriately, on the other hand, is important.)

CONCLUSION

With regard to stress and IBS, people should be aware of new medications that are being developed that will act as CRF antagonists, meaning they will block this aspect of the stress response (elevated CRF levels) in the gut. Currently, a number of researchers and pharmaceutical companies are conducting research in this area, and we can expect to see public announcements of studies related to it in the months and years ahead.

If the drugs being developed work as intended, they may prove useful in their ability to block the bacterial overgrowth that otherwise results from the slowing of the small intestine cleansing waves during increased CRF production. It still remains to be seen whether such drugs will be able to accomplish this. What is most important in treating IBS is not reducing factors that inhibit these cleansing waves, but actually stimulating them to do their job more effectively while at the same time eliminating the bacterial overgrowth that is the primary cause of IBS. This is something that my colleagues and I are able to do quickly and effectively using the Cedars-Sinai treatment protocol, which you will read about in Part Two.

CHAPTER 4

Guess Who's
Coming to Dinner
Food Poisoning and Parasites

When Francis was thirty-five years old, he vacationed in Hawaii. At the time, he was perfectly healthy, with no abnormal bowel habits. During the third day of his vacation, after grabbing a quick bite to eat at a fast food eatery, he experienced feelings of indigestion but ignored them, eager to enjoy some more time on the beach. The next day, however, Francis woke up feeling nauseous and had to rush to the bathroom to vomit. This was followed by diarrhea that ruined the rest of his vacation. Instead of being able to enjoy himself, he was forced to remain close to his hotel room, going to the bathroom eight to ten times a day.

Francis thought his symptoms were from food poisoning from his meal at the fast food eatery. Eventually, his diarrhea symptoms tapered off, but soon after he returned home, he began to experience other gastrointestinal disturbances. Primarily, at first, he was bothered by bloating and abdominal distension. Then he experienced a chronic pattern of bloating on a daily basis accompanied by alternating patterns of constipation and diarrhea.

When Francis first came to me for help with his symptoms, he was forty-five years old and had endured his symptoms for ten years. Nothing he had tried prior to consulting with me had given him more than temporary, fleeting relief. Listening to Francis explain his symptoms, I knew that he was suffering from IBS. When follow-up diagnostic tests failed to confirm any other condition, I told Francis what he had.

He said, "It was my damned trip to Hawaii! Everything was fine until I ate at that eatery. Ever since then, my gastrointestinal tract's been a mess!"

Sally, another of my patients, was exposed to the amoeba parasite after she drank water during a trip to Latin America. Soon thereafter, she developed chronic bowel complaints that she suffered from for years. Eventually, the amoeba was discovered and treated, but her bowel symptoms did not fully improve. Subsequent diagnostic tests, which were repeated more than once, revealed that the amoeba was gone, yet her bowel symptoms continued unabated. When Sally first consulted with me, she was fifty-five years old and had endured her symptoms—which were also due to IBS—for seven years. Like Francis, she distinctly recalled her trip as the time her symptoms began. "If only I'd avoided drinking the water!" Sally said ruefully. Fortunately, today Francis and Sally are both symptom-free after following the IBS protocol that you will read about in Part Two. What Francis and Sally have in common with as many as 20 percent of all IBS patients is that their symptoms were preceded by an acute episode of food poisoning (Francis) or traveler's diarrhea (Sally).

Investigators in Europe conducted the initial research that suggested that food poisoning and certain types of parasitic infection (primarily amoeba, *Cryptosporidium parvum*, and giardia, each of which can be contracted by drinking contaminated water) may precipitate what is known as "post-infectious IBS" (IBS that occurs after an episode of food poisoning or parasitic infection). They discovered this by examining patients who had documented cases of food poisoning, also known as acute gastroenteritis (in some cases, the food poisoning was so severe that the patients had to be admitted to the hospital), or acute infectious diarrhea.

None of these patients were found to have IBS at the time. But later, well after the incriminating infection (food poisoning or parasite) had either resolved itself or been successfully treated (determined by stool samples showing that the infectious organism was no longer present), the patients went on to develop IBS. In all, the researchers discovered that 7 to 31 percent of patients with either acute gastroenteritis or acute infectious diarrhea subsequently developed IBS.

When the researchers presented their initial findings, they were met with a certain degree of skepticism by some IBS specialists, who still considered IBS to be primarily a psychological condition. While not rejecting the findings outright, these specialists questioned whether the symptoms the patients developed after suffering with food poisoning or parasites were really those of IBS. Perhaps, they suggested, the actual reason for the patients' ongoing symptoms was that the infectious agent had somehow damaged the gastrointestinal tract and the damage had yet to heal.

To address such questions, the researchers conducted a follow-up study, which they published in 2002. In this study, they observed that 57 percent of the people who developed IBS after initially suffering from food poisoning still met all the Rome criteria for IBS six years later. This clearly indicated that their symptoms were indeed consistent with chronic IBS. Food poisoning is very common, yet not everyone who experiences food poisoning develops IBS. Conversely, could most of the IBS cases have been caused by this type of acute infection? Unfortunately, the answer to that question currently remains unanswered, because most people who experience food poisoning, which usually resolves itself within a week or so, never see a doctor for their problem.

What we now know is that a significant percentage of these people do go on to develop IBS, and it remains possible that many cases of IBS may be secondary to food poisoning or certain types of parasitic infection. But the only way to answer this question would be for every known case of food poisoning to be tracked at its onset to see what happens after it resolves. That would be difficult to achieve.

In addition, there are still many IBS specialists who continue to reject the causal link between food poisoning and IBS. Although they accept the possibility that food poisoning causes IBS, they label such incidents as a subcategory of IBS—that is, post-infectious IBS. Their argument in support of their position is that, among a sampling of one hundred IBS patients, perhaps twenty of them can be identified as post-infectious IBS patients, while the remaining eighty cannot. Still, the significance of cases of IBS that are subsequent to food poisoning should not be overlooked. For example, in my own practice, when I ask IBS patients if they can remember what I have termed a "heralding episode" or "heralding event," 20 to 30 percent of any group of patients state that they can recall exactly when their IBS started. In some cases, they remember the specific date it began. They tell that

Risk Factors for Developing Post-Infectious IBS

Although it remains unclear as to whether all cases of IBS stem from food poisoning and/or parasitic infection, more than ten years of scientific research have clearly established that a significant percentage of IBS patients first developed their symptoms after they were exposed to such heralding events. Here are some of the most important factors you must know to minimize your risk of developing post-infectious IBS.

➤ *Campylobacter*—Of all infectious agents (bacteria, parasites, and viruses), this bacterium has the greatest likelihood of initiating post-infectious IBS. As it is primarily transmitted through contaminated food or fecal-oral transmission, you can drastically minimize your risk of being exposed to *Campylobacter* by taking care to avoid food poisoning (see *Tips For Avoiding Food Poisoning* on page 44).

➤ **The severity of the heralding event**—Research has also discovered that the intensity of the heralding event, such as the duration and severity of traveler's diarrhea, has a direct correlation to the likelihood of post-infectious IBS. For example, someone whose diarrhea symptoms last for two weeks or more is at a significantly greater risk for IBS than someone whose symptoms last for only a day or two.

that they remember eating at a particular restaurant or recall a trip that resulted in food poisoning. Ever since those heralding events, they report, they've suffered with IBS. In every case, the heralding event they recall was also very pronounced: it was the worst diarrhea of their life, or they remember that there was blood in their stool, or something equally significant and dramatic.

Research into post-infectious IBS and its link to heralding events such as food poisoning or parasitic infection continues. Because of the results, which began to be reported in 1994, researchers started to investigate different types of bacteria and other infectious agents to discover if there was a single agent that was causing post-infectious IBS, just as we now know that the *H. pylori* bacteria is the most common cause of ulcers. If that were the case, it might be possible to vaccinate against the agent or at least disrupt its ability to initiate IBS. But

> The degree of vomiting during the heralding event—Following exposure to food poisoning, the less one vomits, the more likely one is to develop post-infectious IBS. This is especially true when lack of vomiting is accompanied by diarrhea. Certain food-poisoning bacteria produce vomiting, others diarrhea. It appears that the bacteria that principally affect the small bowel and colon are connected with IBS, and not those that principally affect the stomach.

> Gender—In a study published in 2002, it was found that women who got food poisoning were much more likely to develop post-infectious IBS after they experienced food poisoning compared with men. The reason for this is not yet known, but this may explain why more women have IBS than men. In the meantime, if you are a woman, you should especially take good care to avoid food poisoning.

> Age—Overall, young adults are more prone to post-infectious IBS following a heralding event than are older people.

> Stress level—Even though it's now been shown that IBS is not a stress or psychological disorder, research appears to indicate that a person's stress level or psychological state at the time of the food poisoning may affect progression of post-infectious IBS.

it turned out that this isn't the case. Instead, researchers have found that infections from a number of bacteria can lead to IBS, including *Campylobacter, Salmonella,* and *Shigella,* as well as parasites such as amoeba and giardia. In some cases, certain types of viruses have also been shown to cause post-infectious IBS. In 2004, a study was published showing that, among bacteria, *Campylobacter* was found to be most likely to cause post-infectious IBS. *Campylobacter* is primarily contracted from food poisoning and tends to make most people very sick.

Despite the large amount of research conducted in Europe since 1994 that established a strong link between infectious organisms and post-infectious IBS, until recently most IBS researchers and physicians in the United States continued to operate under the supposition that IBS is primarily caused by stress and that its symptoms are "all in a patient's head." In fact, as of this writing, in the United States the first investigations into post-infectious IBS have only been in the last year. U.S. physicians, scientists, and researchers who specialize in IBS are more than a decade behind their European colleagues when it comes to examining this association.

A dramatic example of how food poisoning can cause post-infectious IBS occurred in May 2000 in the Canadian town of Walkerton, Ontario, and was described by a highly respected researcher, Dr. Stephen Collins. Due to heavy rainfall that caused runoff from farmlands, fertilizer and other contaminants ended up in the town's wells that provided its water supply. As a result, approximately 2,300 of the town's 4,500 residents experienced acute food poisoning after drinking the water. Of these, six people died and another sixty-five had to be hospitalized. Three years later, approximately 1,000 of the 2,300 people who experienced acute gastroenteritis still suffered from chronic gastrointestinal tract disorders consistent with post-infectious IBS. That's nearly 50 percent of the population in question. Such an incident makes the link between food poisoning and other heralding events and post-infectious IBS very difficult to ignore.

INFLAMMATION AND POST-INFECTIOUS IBS

In 2000, European researchers took our understanding of how food poisoning can lead to post-infectious IBS to the next level. They accomplished this by taking biopsies of the rectums of IBS patients known to have had food poisoning as the cause of their IBS. Their research showed that there were increased white blood cell counts in the lining of the rectums of patients with post-infectious IBS. This indicates that even after the heralding event is resolved and the food-poisoning bacteria are gone, inflammation remains in the rectum.

While the elevated white blood cell counts in the rectum are higher than normal, the degree of inflammation is so modest as to appear inconsequential to most pathologists. It is possible that the cell count elevation is due to the fact that these patients continue to suffer from diarrhea months and years after the initial heralding event, and that is what is irritating the rectum. In a follow-up study, IBS patients whose symptoms were not deemed to be post-infectious also showed elevated white blood cell counts, although not to the same extent as that exhibited by post-infectious IBS patients. This could be because the non-post-infectious IBS patients included people whose IBS symptoms were constipation predominant. This might possibly have skewed the findings to indicate a higher elevation in post-infectious IBS patients than was actually the case. This elevated white blood cell count in the rectal lining is now becoming the basis for a new set of studies looking at the consequences of inflammation in IBS.

In people who experience food poisoning but do not develop post-infectious IBS, the body initiates an inflammatory response, including elevated white blood cell counts, in order to attack and rid itself of the invading microorganism. Once this is accomplished, the inflammatory response is stopped and the body returns to normal. This is what happens with the majority of people who experience acute gastroenteritis—the inflammatory response does its job and they completely recover.

Why complete recovery does not occur in people who then develop post-infectious IBS is a question still in need of answers. There are a number of possibilities that could account for this, including a person's genetics, immune response (responding too fast or too slow to the invading pathogens), the type of bacteria and/or toxins, and other factors. Although determining which factors play a role remains an important focus for our better overall understanding of IBS, equally important is the now-established fact that heralding events such as acute gastroenteritis account for a high percentage of all IBS cases. Therefore, it makes good sense to take measures to avoid food poisoning in the first place.

COPING WITH FOOD POISONING

Before researchers and physicians were aware that food poisoning could lead to post-infectious IBS, it was commonly thought that the symptoms of food poisoning, especially diarrhea, should be allowed to run their course so that the body could rid itself of the offending toxin or pathogen.

In the majority of cases, this approach leads to a complete resolution of food-poisoning symptoms with no further problems. However, knowing what we do now about the link between food poisoning and post-infectious IBS, "letting nature take its course" may not always be the wisest approach. This is especially true of diarrhea that lasts for

Tips for Avoiding Food Poisoning

Food poisoning is becoming an increasingly common occurrence due to the fact that people are traveling and eating out more than they used to. Statistics show that 12 percent of all travelers will experience food poisoning as soon as they leave their home city or town. It makes no difference whether they travel to Philadelphia or Mexico: 12 percent of all travelers are guaranteed to get food poisoning.

For travelers who do travel outside of the United States, especially to Third-World countries, the percentage is much higher, perhaps as high as 50 percent.

Symptoms of food poisoning can vary, ranging from onset within 30 to 60 minutes after eating (usually in cases of chemical contaminants in food) to up to 12 to 48 hours in cases of bacterial food poisoning. Many cases of diarrhea are due to food poisoning, although this may not be recognized at the time. Other symptoms of food poisoning include nausea, stomach pain, vomiting, and, in very severe cases, collapse and shock from dehydration.

To minimize your risk of contracting food poisoning, do the following:

➢ Avoid eating at street vendors, which are common in foreign countries.

➢ Avoid salad bars where food can be set out all day and exposed to a host of potentially food-poisoning microorganisms.

➢ Heat, Heat, Heat. Hot food is safe. Room temperature is an absolute no.

➢ Avoid eating raw fish, including sushi.

more than a day or two because, as we discussed earlier, the longer the initial period of diarrhea lasts, the more likely a person is to have his or her food-poisoning symptoms eventually progress to post-infectious IBS. If we can shorten the period of diarrhea related to food poisoning, we will be able to reduce the number of people who go on to develop IBS because of it.

The most common method used by people to treat their diarrhea is an over-the-counter drug such as Imodium. While such drugs can bring a certain degree of relief, all they are doing is masking the diarrhea symptoms, not addressing their root cause—the offending bacte-

> ➢ When dining out, select restaurants that have a reputation for cleanliness. Code violations for restaurants that violate good sanitary standards are often posted in local newspapers.

> ➢ When eating poultry that has been frozen, be sure that it is fully thawed before cooking to minimize the risk of salmonella poisoning. For the same reason, also avoid eating raw eggs.

> ➢ At home, wash all fruits and vegetables thoroughly before eating. A variety of nontoxic food detergents are now available for this purpose, as well. You can find them at your local health food store.

> ➢ When traveling, especially to Third-World countries, avoid eating uncooked vegetables, including salads, as these foods are often sprayed and washed with local water. All vegetable dishes should be cooked and served hot.

> ➢ Peel the skins of all fruits before you eat them. If you can peel it, you can eat it. If not, forget it.

> ➢ Also avoid the use of ice cubes, including those added to beverages. Travelers forget that ice cubes are often made with local water.

> ➢ As much as possible, drink brand-name bottled water, and use the same water when brushing your teeth. Also be sure that the water bottle is properly sealed before you open it. If bottled water is unavailable, you can use iodine tablets to treat the water before you use it.

> ➢ When bathing or showering while traveling, avoid getting water in your mouth.

ria. For this reason, studies are now underway to examine the efficacy of using antibiotics during times of acute gastroenteritis. This is not an official medical recommendation at this time, but depending on the studies' results it may become so in the future. At the same time, some pharmaceutical companies are currently investigating the use of antibiotic drugs as a prophylactic (preventive) measure for protecting against food poisoning. I believe that in the near future, under certain circumstances and depending on what regions of the world travelers intend to visit, the use of such preventive antibiotics may, in fact, be medically recommended.

A good example of such a drug is rifaximin (Xifaxan), which is being marketed in the United States by the pharmaceutical company Salix Pharmaceuticals.

Rifaximin is very effective for both preventing and treating traveler's diarrhea and is approved by the FDA for this purpose. One of the reasons rifaximin is so appropriate for food poisoning is because it is a 99.6 percent non-absorbed antibiotic, meaning that instead of moving into the bloodstream and other parts of the body as many antibiotics and other drugs do, rifaximin remains in the gastrointestinal tract where it protects against and targets the invading bacteria known to cause traveler's diarrhea. Recently, rifaximin was shown to reduce not only the length but also the intensity of an acute attack of traveler's diarrhea (the length was reduced by 50 percent). Because of this, rifaximin is now being tested to determine its usefulness in preventing IBS altogether by attacking the disease at its origin—the acute food-poisoning illness. The results are likely to be very promising. If rifaximin works in this way, it will markedly improve our ability to reduce the instances of IBS and more effectively treat it when it does develop.

One of the other reasons why it's important to minimize the duration of acute gastroenteritis may involve how food-poisoning bacteria in the gastrointestinal tract interfere with the cleansing wave of the small intestine. We'll be discussing this aspect of IBS in the next chapter. For now, suffice it to say that when this cleansing wave of motility becomes disturbed, it allows overgrowth of the bacteria associated with chronic IBS, even after the food poisoning has resolved.

Research has shown that these bacteria can affect the cleansing-wave action of the small intestine. Studies in Europe showed that *Campylobacter* disrupts the muscle and nerve connections of the small intestines.

Currently, I am working with my colleagues at Cedars-Sinai conducting research to determine whether the toxin produced by *Campylobacter* completely disrupts the cleansing wave by paralyzing the muscle and nerve connections, thus setting the stage for IBS.

Like all other species, bacteria are primarily concerned with their own survival and propagation. They accomplish both by colonizing their host, or the body of the patient. There, they multiply and then pass themselves on in stool, giving themselves a chance to infect patient number two. In order to do this, the bacteria need to stop the small intestine from cleaning itself out. In some people, this effect on small intestinal movement is only temporary, but in others, the effects may be permanent, thus setting the stage for bacterial proliferation and the chronic symptoms of IBS. Based on the routine clinical success I am having in improving IBS in my patients by addressing bacterial overgrowth, I believe that this bacterial process is the primary cause of IBS.

GOOD BACTERIA, BAD BACTERIA?
EXAMINING THE FACTS

These days, given their popularity, no discussion of the relationship between bacteria overgrowth and IBS can avoid mention of so-called "good" bacteria, also known as probiotics, and their potential benefits as an aid against so-called "bad" bacteria. Many of my patients ask me about this, and I tell them there really is no such thing as "good" and "bad" bacteria in the gastrointestinal tract. The concept of "good bacteria" was coined by the companies that manufacture probiotics. I don't mean to imply that these products cannot be useful at times; I have had some patients tell me that after they used probiotics their IBS symptoms improved. I can't argue with that.

At the same time, IBS, as well as the health of the gastrointestinal tract in general, is far too complex to support a simple claim that certain types of bacteria will solve the problem. As an example, consider the common bacteria *E. coli*. Most people are well aware of how pathogenic strains of *E. coli* can cause serious gastrointestinal problems. Every time there is an outbreak of food poisoning at a fast food restaurant, it is the dreaded *E. coli*. What most people don't realize is that non-pathogenic strains of *E. coli* are some of the best bacteria for maintaining the health of the lining of the intestines, yet no manufacturer is going to market those strains. In the normal gut, *E. coli* is one of the most common bacteria; bad things happen only when a special toxic strain is in the food. Still, this fear of *E. coli* prevents manufacturers from making any probiotics with this type of bacteria.

The two most popular forms of probiotics are *Lactobacillus acidophilus* and *Bifidobacterium bifidum*. Both have been shown to exist in lesser amounts in patients with IBS compared with healthy people when stool samples from both groups are tested. Proponents of such bacteria seized on such findings as evidence that IBS and other gastrointestinal disorders are due, at least in part, to deficiencies of these types of probiotics. If this was the only problem caused by IBS, then supplementing with these types of probiotics should do much to reverse symptoms. Unfortunately, the research into this area does not bear this out. One recent double-blind study conducted by Dr. Eamonn Quigley, for instance, found that there were no measurable improvements among IBS patients who were given *Lactobacillus acidophilus*, but there was some improvement among patients who were given *Bifidobacterium*.

In addition, other studies also indicate that probiotic supplements may not always be safe. There have been case reports of children who were given large doses of *Lactobacillus acidophilus* to help treat their diarrhea who suffered from negative side effects. In one case, a child developed endocarditis (infection of the heart valve) as a result of overconsumption of *Lactobacillus acidophilus*. There have also been reported cases of blood infection in people who consumed too much probiotic.

This doesn't mean that such bacteria have no benefit. The real question concerning bacteria is not whether they are "good" or "bad," but where in the body they are located. As in real estate, when it comes to so-called good and bad bacteria, the most important issue is "location, location, location." If the bacteria are where they are supposed to be in the body and are doing what they are supposed to do, then they are okay. But if they migrate into the wrong place, then they can create problems. For example, *E. coli* in the stool is perfectly okay, but if it migrates into the bloodstream and gets into the urine to cause a urinary tract infection, it is potentially very dangerous. In another example, bacteria migrating into the small intestine can create problems, as so often happens in cases of IBS.

At the same time, there is no question that certain types of bacteria (assuming they are not overconsumed), such as *Lactobacillus acidophilus* and *Bifidobacterium bifidum*, can have beneficial effects on the health of the gastrointestinal tract. One study from Europe showed that these two bacteria can, in fact, increase the cleansing-wave activity of the small intestine, which may be beneficial in IBS. The problem lies with our inability to understand the beneficial effects of bacteria acting together, because they are too complex.

At any given time, there is interplay between 300 and 500 different types of bacteria in the gastrointestinal tract. That's how many species of bacteria are found in human stool; in fact, the bacteria compose 50 percent of total stool weight. Therefore, it is unlikely that one type of bacteria alone, or even in combination with five or ten other types of bacteria, can compensate for the effects of 300 to 500 bacteria. The gut bacterial composition is an infinitely complex mixture of sym-

Fast Facts About Bacteria and the Human Body

➢ Bacteria are one of the oldest living life forms on Earth.

➢ There are far more bacteria cells in the human body than there are human cells.

➢ Bacteria are often complex, in terms of their ability to adjust to their environment.

➢ Half the total weight of all stool in the colon is made up of bacteria.

➢ At any given time, 300 to 500 different types of bacteria are interacting in the human gastrointestinal tract.

➢ Scientists have so far been able to culture approximately only 20 percent of these types of bacteria. Currently, we do not know what the remaining 80 percent of bacteria in the gastrointestinal tract grow on, so culturing them is impossible.

➢ Each human has his or her own fingerprint of types and quantities of bacteria. This fingerprint was likely determined at a very young age, when the immune system was figuring out what was already in the body (therefore, don't react to it) and what was not (therefore, if it ever comes in, we must get rid of it).

➢ Studies have shown that taking an antibiotic will disrupt the fingerprint of bacteria of a person, but after a short period of time, the exact fingerprint of types and numbers of bacteria will return.

biotic bacteria, and altering one or two in this large number seems unlikely to be a curative treatment for any gastrointestinal disease.

A WORD ABOUT PARASITES

As we discussed at the beginning of this chapter, certain types of parasites, such as amoeba (*Entamoeba*) and giardia, can also cause post-infectious IBS. Some health specialists consider parasitic infection to be a more common (yet undiagnosed) condition than many doctors and patients realize. Some experts estimate that as many as 60 percent of all Americans are infected by parasites at some point in their lives.

The symptoms of parasitic infection usually appear within 72 to 120 hours following exposure. Symptoms include diarrhea (which can be explosive and/or watery), constipation, pronounced fatigue, nausea, stomach cramping, and vomiting, most of which are similar to IBS symptoms. Therefore, when treating IBS patients, it is important to consider whether or not parasites might be a culprit. If they are, then treating the parasite may resolve the problem. In order to minimize risk of parasitic infection, follow the same tips for avoiding food poisoning provided earlier. Also don't drink water from rivers or streams during hiking and camping trips, and don't eat raw or undercooked meat or fish.

Being around pets or other animals can also increase the risk of parasitic infection. However, the types of parasites that can be contracted from animals, such as hookworms, nematodes, and pinworms, do not cause the inflammation associated with IBS.

Nonetheless, I have had a few of my IBS patients tell me they believed their IBS symptoms were due to parasites they got from their pets even though testing showed that no such parasites were present. If you suspect you suffer from parasitic infection, see your doctor, who can schedule the proper tests for you.

CONCLUSION

Based on more than a decade of research demonstrating the link between acute gastroenteritis and post-infectious IBS, it is becoming increasingly clear that IBS can be precipitated by a case of acute gastroenteritis. This chapter has provided information on how this occurs and how to prevent acute gastroenteritis. How food poisoning triggers IBS is not known. There is some evidence that food poisoning may damage small bowel movement in a way that may set the stage for IBS. The next few chapters will explore new developments of how normal colon bacteria can cause IBS by excessively colonizing the small bowel, which is due to a failure of small intestinal cleansing contractions between meals.

CHAPTER 5

The New Culprit:
Bacterial Overgrowth

In order for you to fully understand why my colleagues at Cedars-Sinai and I are convinced that the primary cause of IBS is bacterial overgrowth, let's take a look at how our understanding of IBS has evolved.

Earlier, we discussed the Rome criteria, which are still used as a diagnostic tool by most physicians who treat IBS. When the Rome criteria were developed, bloating, abdominal distension, and flatulence (gas) were excluded from the main criteria for IBS and designated as minor. However, prior to the Rome criteria, the research that led to the development of the Manning criteria showed that bloating and abdominal distension were significant features of IBS. However, because no one at that time knew how to treat or explain bloating, the experts who developed the Rome criteria relegated bloating to the list of symptoms considered minor criteria. The Rome experts instead focused on constipation, diarrhea, and abdominal pain as the primary symptoms of IBS. In part, this may have been due to anticipated studies to test treatment of constipation, diarrhea, and abdominal pain with new drugs targeting the serotonin receptor (see Chapter 2).

Further confusing the situation were studies conducted in the 1970s and 1980s, which tried to determine whether or not bloating and distension were actually major symptoms of IBS. Most participants in these studies reported having both of these symptoms, but neither were found upon examination. At best, the examiners found modest protrusions of the stomach, not serious protrusion as might be caused by bowel obstruction. Nonetheless, test subjects continued to insist that as the day progressed their bloating increased and their stomachs became more distended.

Around this time, researchers also began to explore whether or not flatulence was a major symptom of IBS. Again, many IBS patients reported that it was, stating that they frequently passed gas, that it had a foul odor, or that they had gas buildup that they had trouble passing, causing their stomachs to become distended. Again, there were no conclusive findings; the researchers remained uncertain about what role these factors played in IBS. Then, in 1980, the research of Dr. Whitehead was published, showing that most IBS patients experienced more sensitivity to pain in the rectum and intestinal tract compared with non-IBS patients. At this point, the researchers concluded that IBS patients didn't really have gas and distension to any significant degree, but just felt as if they did because of their hypersensitiv-

Bloating, Distension, and Flatulence: The Complaints Doctors Hate to Hear

Although bloating, abdominal distension, and/or flatulence are quite common, they rank among the complaints most likely to make your physician privately groan. This does not mean that your doctor is not sympathetic to your problems, but that doctors hate to hear such complaints because, until now, there was very little that they could do for them. While there are various drugs advertised on television (just watch the evening news) that claim to treat such problems, they actually do not. Take drugs like simethicone, for example, which is widely advertised as being able to reduce gas symptoms. The truth is that virtually no one who uses such products experiences any kind of relief. All that these products do is break the gas bubbles; they do not reduce the amount of gas in your system. Unlike other gastrointestinal symptoms such as constipation and diarrhea, both of which are relatively easy to treat, bloating, distension, and flatulence are much harder to treat and are therefore a source of great frustration for physicians and patients alike.

ity to pain. However, the researchers had very little real data to support this conclusion.

This situation began to change when researchers in Europe, Lea and colleagues, developed an electronic belt that could be worn for twenty-four hours, which measured the continuous girth of the stomach. The results showed that IBS patients truly *did* have far more distention than normal. Though they awoke with stomachs that were relatively normal, over the course of the day and night, as they ate their meals, their stomachs became increasingly distended, and then, during sleep, regressed back to normal by the next morning. This research showed that this abnormal distention was a typical pattern among IBS patients.

Around this same time, additional research by Dr. T. S. King also demonstrated higher-than-normal levels of gas produced among IBS patients compared with healthy people. The average human produces many liters of gas each day. However, most people do not pass all of the gas out of their rectums, but reabsorb it and expel it as they breathe. Prior to King's research, researchers in the 1970s and 1980s were unable to detect any significant difference in rectal gas expulsion between IBS patients and healthy controls. This was because they didn't account for the fermenting gas that was getting reabsorbed and expelled in the breath. King, therefore, placed IBS patients and controls in sealed chambers, where he measured all bacterial fermenting gases that were expelled from both normal breathing and through the rectum. He found that the IBS patients produced approximately five times as much gas of a bacterial source compared with the control group. Though King proved that IBS patients did produce far more gas from a bacterial source than normal, he concluded that the reason was that they had too much bacteria in the colon.

King's research was followed by a study group from Japan (Koide and colleagues), which took x-rays of the stomachs of IBS patients and compared them to x-rays of stomachs of test subjects in a control group. Koide's group discovered that IBS patients had significantly greater amounts of gas in their small intestines.

Based on these three studies, which showed that IBS patients overall have excessive bloating of the stomach, produce far greater levels of gas from a bacterial source than healthy people do, and have excessive accumulations of such gas in the small intestine, my colleagues and

I at Cedars-Sinai's GI Motility Program reasoned that the primary cause of IBS more than likely was excessive bacteria in the small intestine.

Even after our research validated our hypothesis, we still faced an uphill battle in terms of gaining acceptance for the primary link between bacterial overgrowth and IBS from the majority of physicians who treat IBS, a situation that still exists to this day. The reason for this resistance, in addition to the still-held belief that IBS is primarily a psychological condition, is that IBS continues to be a diagnosis of exclusion.

As we discussed earlier, a diagnosis of exclusion means that the diagnosis was made only if nothing else appears to be wrong, that is if no diagnostic tests show any results. Here's how the diagnosis of exclusion works when it comes to the refusal of physicians and researchers to accept bacterial overgrowth as the primary cause of IBS: While bacterial overgrowth has been shown to occur in significantly higher levels among IBS patients than in non-IBS patients, those who believe the diagnosis of exclusion claim that signs of IBS can't show up on a test, so the bacterial overgrowth cannot indicate IBS.

How do we know that IBS is *not* a diagnosis of exclusion? To understand how, consider again the relationship between the bacteria *H. pylori* and peptic ulcers. Although the original researchers whose work proved that *H. pylori* is the principal cause of peptic ulcers were roundly criticized and ridiculed when they first presented their findings in the 1980s (at which time peptic ulcers were also seen as being primarily due to stress), today it is accepted that the researchers were right. Therefore, to say that evidence of bacterial overgrowth in people with IBS means that they don't have IBS is exactly akin to saying that evidence of *H. pylori* in people with peptic ulcers means they don't have peptic ulcers either; they have *H. pylori* disease. In the latter case, mainstream physicians and researchers today would dismiss this. Yet the diagnosis of exclusion, which resists identifying bacterial overgrowth as the cause of IBS, continues to be debated. This book was written to help change this perception.

BREATH TESTS CONFIRM
BACTERIAL OVERGROWTH IN IBS PATIENTS

Physicians have used breath tests for quite some time, but my colleagues and I at Cedars-Sinai (including my mentor, Dr. Henry C. Lin) were the first to use them in a published study that confirmed the IBS-bacterial overgrowth link. This came about in the 1990s, as we began noticing how often IBS patients told their physicians that their condition improved when they were given antibiotics. One example of this was Susan, a thirty-seven-year-old woman who had suffered with IBS symptoms for six years. After having a root canal, Susan was placed on a course of antibiotics for two weeks. During that time, she told her primary-care physician that her IBS symptoms had greatly improved for two months, only to flare up again. Susan wondered if there was a connection between the antibiotics and the temporary improvement in her IBS symptoms, but her physician dismissed the idea as a simple coincidence.

Based on our knowledge of greater incidence of bacterial overgrowth among IBS patients, as well as reports such as Susan's where IBS symptoms significantly improved during antibiotic treatments, my colleagues and I began to suspect that not only was bacterial overgrowth a potential cause of IBS, but that the proper course of antibiotic treatment might be effective. We began to notice how many IBS patients tested positive for elevated levels of bacteria during breath tests at our center, and also how many of those patients reported that their IBS symptoms improved when they used antibiotics. In many cases, the symptoms improved to the point where the patients were feeling normal again.

We decided to study the IBS patients who came to our center for breath tests, to determine how many tested positive for bacterial overgrowth. In the first study, we screened over 200 patients; 76 percent tested positive for bacterial overgrowth. These patients were then treated with antibiotics, and afterward returned for follow-up breath tests. Much of the patients' bacterial overgrowth either significantly reduced or returned to normal levels, and in each case, there was also a corresponding, remarkable improvement in their IBS symptoms. We published the results of this study in the *American Journal of Gastroenterology* in 2000. When this study was published, the results were considered controversial, and many researchers criticized it for not being a controlled double-blind study. In addition, some researchers questioned whether the results were due to the fact that Cedars-Sinai's GI Motility Program receives visits from patients who are sick, with the bacterial overgrowth simply being a result of their illness. Finally, some researchers questioned our findings, saying we had not proved that the bacteria were in the small intestine because we had not cultured them from the gut. Whenever bacteria are believed to be responsible for a condition, the way to prove it is to culture the bacteria from a sample from the site of the condition.

We took this last criticism very seriously, and we decided to study the gut bacteria of IBS patients. We discussed this with some of the nation's top experts in infection and bacteria, including normal gut bacteria, but were discouraged because at the time there was no method for growing 80 percent of the 400 species of normal bacteria that reside in the small intestine, the site of the bacteria associated with IBS. To culture only the remaining 20 percent would not provide enough information. Furthermore, there currently was no way to collect samples of bacteria from the small intestine without contaminating the instrument used to collect them as it passes through the mouth, throat, and so forth. And, even if collection without contamination were possible, the gut bacteria cannot live in the presence of oxygen, and would immediately die once they were exposed to oxygen when removed from the patient.

Given such problems, my colleagues and I instead decided to repeat the breath tests as a double-blind study. We recruited patients from the general community instead of from our clinic, and we conducted breath tests that were completely blinded, meaning that we did not know if the patients had bacterial overgrowth or not. Their breath was collected and sealed, and then the patients were randomly given neomycin (an antibiotic) or a placebo that they took for ten days. Within a week to ten days after they completed their course of antibiotic or placebo treatments, the patients returned for another breath test and a reevaluation of their symptoms. The test results revealed that 84 percent exhibited bacterial overgrowth based on the breath test. The patients who then received neomycin had a 35 percent improvement of their symptoms, compared with only 11 percent in the placebo group. This difference was statistically significant. Even more remarkably, among the patients whose breath tests returned to normal as a result of using neomycin, approximately 75 percent also experienced improvement in their IBS symptoms, which was one of the highest improvement rates ever demonstrated in IBS patients.

This was based on a composite score of the commonly accepted symptoms associated with IBS, such as constipation, diarrhea, and abdominal pain. We published this study in 2003 in the *American Journal of Gastroenterology.*

Although culturing is difficult, two studies, conducted by Drs. Simren and Robson, found that 12 percent of IBS patients have colon bacteria in excess of 100,000 per milliliter all the way up to the duodenum, the highest part of the upper bowel. While the 12 percent in this study is not the same as the 84 percent found in our study, the difference is that the duodenum is the part of the gastrointestinal tract farthest away from the colon (source of bacteria). In addition, those who tested positive for bacterial overgrowth in the duodenum also had the worst IBS symptoms, suggesting that the closer we get to the colon, the higher the percentage of bacterial overgrowth. The 12 percent finding, in other words, is really the bare-minimum percentage of bacterial overgrowth detectable among IBS patients.

Although breath tests had already been in use for a number of decades prior to the tests we conducted, my colleagues and I at Cedars-Sinai were the first researchers to use them in the clinical management of IBS. Our studies, as well as later studies conducted by other researchers, have demonstrated the fact that bacterial overgrowth is the primary factor in cases of IBS. The improvement IBS patients demonstrate when they follow the Cedars-Sinai protocol for treating IBS by normalizing bacterial levels cannot be disputed. This improvement is something that we are now achieving on a routine basis.

WHAT CAUSES BACTERIAL OVERGROWTH?

The human body is designed to prevent bacterial overgrowth and has various mechanisms for doing so. To keep the wrong kind of bacteria out of the gastrointestinal tract, the immune system identifies and attacks invading bacteria as well as other pathogens, such as viruses and fungi. To prevent bacterial overgrowth in the small intestine, the primary defenses are stomach acid, which kills bacteria that enters through the mouth (with a few exceptions, such as *H. pylori,* which can survive stomach acid), and bile juices secreted by the gallbladder and pancreas.

How Breath Tests Are Performed

Breath tests have been used by physicians as a diagnostic tool for decades. Breath testing itself is very simple, and there are three common ways to perform breath tests as a means of diagnosing bacterial overgrowth—a xylose breath test, a glucose breath test, and a lactulose breath test. Xylose, glucose, and lactulose are all sugars.

The test that we principally use at Cedars-Sinai is the lactulose breath test, because lactulose is the only sugar not absorbed by the body, meaning that it is able to travel all the way through the small intestine, which is approximately 15 feet long. By contrast, glucose, the body's principal energy source, is completely absorbed by the body within the first one or two feet of the gastrointestinal tract; while xylose is less absorbable than glucose, it has varying absorption rates depending on a person's height and body size, making the xylose test difficult to control. Therefore, if you are trying to detect bacteria located in the lower half of the small intestine, only the lactulose test is capable of doing so.

Patients taking this test drink a sample of lactulose syrup. Then, every fifteen minutes over a three-hour period, samples of their breath are collected. Once you drink the lactulose syrup, it quickly comes in contact with the bacteria in the small intestine. The bacteria then eat and digest the lactulose, fermenting it and producing different types of gases—carbon dioxide, hydrogen, methane, and sometimes hydrogen sulfide. Only the hydrogen and methane are detectable in the breath, so they are the gases measured to determine the levels of the various bacteria in the gut.

In healthy people, the largest concentration of bacteria is in the colon. It takes approximately two hours from the time the lactulose syrup is consumed to the time it reaches the colon and starts to be consumed by the bacteria there. This means that healthy people should not experience an increase in bacterial gas production during the breath test until about two hours or more after drinking the sugar.

If the breath test indicates that the bacteria levels are rising within ninety minutes or less, and in concentrations of twenty or more parts per million, that is a strong indication that bacterial overgrowth exists in the small intestine, because the syrup solution reaches the small intestine before it reaches the colon.

An additional point to consider if you decide to have a breath test is the type of instrument your medical practitioner uses. The device that is used most extensively is known as a QuinTron gas chromatograph. For the most accurate reading, I recommend the QuinTron SC, which is capable of measuring both hydrogen and methane, and correcting for possible contamination of the sample by using carbon dioxide from the breath to ensure that the breath samples that are collected are done so correctly. To locate a physician in your area who uses the QuinTron device, contact QuinTron Instrument Company, 3712 West Pierce Street, Milwaukee, WI 53215. Phone: 800–542–4448; Website: www.quintron-usa.com.

In addition, a valve called the ileocecal valve, which is shaped like a little sphincter, prevents bacteria that belong in the colon from moving backward into the small intestine. Then there are the lymphocytes that line the lining of the gastrointestinal tract. Lymphocytes are white blood cells that are an important component of the immune system. They play an essential role in identifying and attacking foreign pathogens. Except for the bone marrow, where most lymphocytes are produced, the lining of the gastrointestinal tract has a higher concentration of lymphocytes than any other part of the body. They prevent bacteria from penetrating the lining of the intestine and traveling to the rest of the body.

Another important mechanism that prevents bacterial overgrowth is a special cleansing action of the small intestine; the cleansing wave. When we are not eating, this cleansing wave is designed to occur every ninety minutes. It is supposed to be deactivated only when we are eating a meal, when the body is digesting food and absorbing the nutrients. Once these are absorbed into the bloodstream, the leftover food particles need to be cleaned out of the small intestine so that the body can be ready for its next meal. The cleaning process begins in the stomach and then moves through the small intestine as the cleansing wave pushes the leftover food particles into the colon for elimination. Ideally, you should have approximately nine cleansing waves of this nature each day.

Researchers have known since 1978 that if you don't have normal cleansing waves throughout the day and night, bacterial overgrowth can occur. In the 1980s, studies were done in which test subjects were given morphine, which inhibits cleansing waves. Over time, these test subjects developed bacterial overgrowth.

Similarly, in the studies my colleagues and I conducted at Cedars-Sinai, we demonstrated that IBS patients with bacterial overgrowth have had on average a 70 percent reduction in cleansing-wave activity when compared with healthy patients.

This evidence ties into the heralding events such as food poisoning that we discussed in Chapter 4. The data that my colleagues and I are compiling strongly indicates that certain food-poisoning toxins significantly inhibit the cleansing wave. This makes sense, because the bacteria that cause food poisoning need to secure a foothold in the small intestine, replicate, and colonize their new environment. The bacteria will need to inactivate the cleansing-wave process so that they don't get expelled. Research in Europe shows that this is exactly what happens with the *Campylobacter* toxin, a very common type of food poison. It disrupts the muscle and nerve connections of the small intestine, stopping the wave, thus allowing the *Campylobacter* bacteria to colonize there. Therefore, if there is no other cause of the cleansing-wave inhibition, future research may confirm that it is due to food poisoning.

METHANE AND HYDROGEN
AND THEIR RELATIONSHIP TO IBS

One of the questions my colleagues and I faced when we published our findings linking bacterial overgrowth to IBS was how those findings explained the various subtypes of IBS. As we discussed in Chapter 2, IBS appears in seemingly opposite ways. Some IBS patients experience frequent diarrhea as an IBS symptom, and little to no constipation (diarrhea-predominant IBS). Others are primarily constipated and experience little to no diarrhea (constipation-predominant IBS). Still others experience constipation and diarrhea in approximately equal measures.

The degree to which an IBS patient experiences constipation or diarrhea is determined, at least in part, by the types of gases produced by the bacteria that have colonized the small intestine. In the breath

Other Factors That Can Cause Bacterial Overgrowth

Although the absence of cleansing waves is known to cause bacterial over-growth, it is vital to consider other known causes. Among them are:

➤ Adhesions on the bowel due to prior abdominal surgery.

➤ Surgery that alters the anatomy of the small intestine.

➤ Endometriosis (abnormal growth of the uterine lining) that extends into the bowel.

➤ Crohn's disease, especially if accompanied by strictures (narrowing of the stomach).

➤ Insufficient production of pancreatic enzymes and/or impaired pancreatic function (often caused by chronic inflammation of the pancreas).

➤ Lack of stomach acid.

➤ AIDS/HIV-related bowel disease.

➤ Aging.

➤ Impaired functioning of the ileocecal valve, which connects the small intestine to the bowel and prevents bacteria, undigested food particles, and other substances in the colon from traveling backward into the small intestine.

tests my colleagues and I conducted, we found higher-than-normal concentrations of two gases—methane and hydrogen—in most of the patients who also tested positive for IBS. Methane and hydrogen are not produced by humans, but by bacteria as part of their fermentation process. We examined close to a thousand IBS patients: in nearly every case, patients whose breath tests showed only higher methane concentrations were constipation predominant. These findings led us to conduct a series of animal studies in which methane was infused into the small intestine. When this was done, transit time in the animals' intestinal tract was reduced by approximately 70 percent, indicating that bowel function slows down in response to methane interacting with the gastrointestinal tract. We concluded that methane is a primary factor responsible for constipation in IBS patients.

In our most recent study, my colleagues and I further demonstrated this by showing that successful treatment of constipation in IBS patients directly depends on the elimination of methane, presumably by eliminating methane-producing bacteria. This is done through the judicious use of antibiotics, which we will discuss in far more detail in Chapter 6. To be sure that the bacteria are really eliminated, a follow-up breath test must be performed. This study showed that constipation will not completely resolve unless the bacteria that produce methane are eliminated.

Interestingly, one way in which methane causes constipation is by causing the bowel to become hyperactive, which my colleagues and I demonstrated in additional studies.

We then reexamined our IBS patients and found that those whose breath tests showed higher concentrations of methane had twice as much small intestine movement as did those whose breath tests showed higher concentrations of hydrogen. However, this movement is counterproductive; instead of moving forward to allow proper elimination of waste products, it moves backward and thus slows down the elimination process.

By contrast, IBS patients with higher concentrations of hydrogen, as opposed to methane, gas in the small intestine experience more diarrhea. However, unlike methane, hydrogen appears not to affect small intestinal physiology, meaning that it doesn't trigger diarrhea symptoms in the same way that methane causes symptoms of constipation. Rather, the degree of diarrhea appears to be related to the quantity of hydrogen-producing bacteria in the small intestine. In addition, studies that my colleagues and I conducted examining IBS patients with fibromyalgia-like symptoms—something I discuss in more detail in Chapter 8—found that patients whose IBS is associated with fibromyalgia also have the highest concentrations of hydrogen levels. Again, this does not mean that the hydrogen is causing the fibromyalgia symptoms, only that the higher the hydrogen levels are, the more bacteria there are, and the sicker these patients tend to be.

In concluding this section, I want to again stress that the bacteria that are producing methane or hydrogen in the small intestine are not necessarily pathogenic or "bad" bacteria. Rather, they are bacteria that should be in the colon but have migrated back into the small intestine because the small bowel cleansing wave is not operating normally. In healthy people, these bacteria can be found in the small intestine, but only in minute, insignificant quantities, and the action of the cleansing waves prevents them from growing beyond those levels.

But if these waves stop, or other factors occur (see page 63), these bacteria start to replicate without being properly eliminated, eventually to the point where IBS can occur.

A UNIFIED THEORY: HOW BACTERIAL OVERGROWTH RELATES TO PREVIOUS THEORIES ABOUT THE CAUSE OF IBS

As I discussed in Chapters 1 to 4, various other theories have been used by physicians and researchers to explain how IBS occurs. Each of those theories can now be better understood, given what we now know about the link between bacterial overgrowth and IBS. For example, the question of IBS subtypes—that is, IBS that is either too fast (diarrhea predominant) or too slow (constipation predominant) can now be explained by the amount of methane that is being produced as a result of bacterial overgrowth in the small intestine.

As Chapter 1 made clear, for many years IBS was considered to be a condition that was primarily caused by psychological factors, especially stress. I don't believe that stress is the cause of IBS, and increasingly, IBS experts across the nation are now coming to that same conclusion. However, recent research has demonstrated that stress can cause CRF (corticotrophin-releasing factor) to increase in the brain (see Chapter 3). Interestingly, when this happens, three things occur in the gastrointestinal tract: The colon empties faster, at times causing diarrhea; the emptying of food from the stomach slows down, causing people to not want to eat; and cleansing waves become inhibited. Therefore, though stress does not cause IBS, the increased CRF that is associated with stress can exacerbate IBS symptoms.

Additionally, future studies may show that food poisoning may herald IBS by causing cleansing-wave inhibition, thus setting the stage for bacterial overgrowth to occur. Because stress already inhibits the cleansing waves, food poisoning occurring at the same time is likely to make matters worse.

Before concluding, let's examine the issue of gut speed and hypersensitivity. Animal studies spanning decades have long demonstrated that bacteria, once they become relocated in the small intestine, can cause the gut to move faster, secrete excessive fluids, and increase the release of a chemical compound known as "Substance P." Substance P is now believed to be the chemical that increases hypersensitivity in the gastrointestinal tract and lowers the pain threshold in the rectum. In addition, when bacterial overgrowth is present in the small intestine, the release of serotonin is also increased. This affirms the belief of IBS researchers who feel that serotonin plays a role in IBS. It definitely does, but the mechanism may be secondary to the bacterial overgrowth itself.

CONCLUSION

What all of this means is that the previous theories related to the cause of IBS were not wrong. In a nutshell, all theories are part of a larger picture that includes food poisoning leading to poor gut-cleansing movements, leading to bacterial overgrowth, leading to substance P release (gut hypersensitivity) and serotonin release (increased speed of the gut/diarrhea) with stress worsening IBS by further inhibiting cleansing waves. A vicious cycle.

In the next part, we will begin to address how to make things better by discussing management strategies.

PART TWO

The IBS Treatment Plan: Putting It All Together

CHAPTER 6

Help at Last:
The Cedars-Sinai Protocol for Treating IBS

Now that you understand how and why bacterial overgrowth is the primary cause of IBS, it's time to learn how to treat IBS most effectively. The goal of your treatment program should be not only to reduce the volume of bacterial overgrowth, but also to eliminate it completely, and then to restore the small intestine's cleansing-wave mechanism. In this way, not only will you resolve your IBS, but you will also prevent its recurrence. I call this comprehensive treatment approach the Cedars-Sinai protocol for treating IBS, because my colleagues and I developed the protocol at the Cedars-Sinai Medical Center in Los Angeles, California.

In this chapter, you will discover how and why the Cedars-Sinai protocol for IBS works, as well as the in-depth screening tests our IBS patients undergo when they first come to my colleagues and me. These tests help to rule out any other underlying conditions. In addition, you will receive diet tips and a one-week menu plan that you can start immediately, which will help to reduce the bacterial load in your gastrointestinal tract, thereby helping to ease your IBS symptoms. Lastly, you will read how the Cedars-Sinai protocol for IBS effectively helped one of my IBS patients, who will recount her successful outcome. Keep in mind that her success story is only one of many.

GETTING STARTED: THE TESTING PHASE

When an IBS patient comes to see me, I first test the patient to determine whether any other factors are contributing to the symptoms. This is something I recommend that all physicians do for patients who complain of IBS-like symptoms, because proper medical screening and diagnostic tests can save lives. Because the clinic I work in is a specialized center for IBS, many of my patients have already undergone such tests before they come to see me, but if they have not, the following are some of the tests I recommend.

Blood Testing

Blood tests are performed to screen for anemia and inflammation. Elevated inflammation levels are indicated by an inflammation marker in the blood called "erythrocyte sedimentation rate" (ESR). Erythrocytes are mature red blood cells, which play a role in transporting oxygen to, and carbon dioxide from, the cells, organs, and tissues, and which also help regulate the acid-alkaline balance of the blood. The ESR test measures the speed at which erythrocytes settle and can help determine if inflammation is present in the body.

Blood tests are also useful in measuring overall blood chemistry, as well as kidney function, and can also indicate other "red flags" for other health imbalances.

Celiac Testing

Celiac disease is a gastrointestinal disorder that can mimic IBS. Its symptoms include faulty digestion of food, malabsorption of nutrients, and diarrhea. Celiac disease is caused by sensitivity to gluten, which is found in wheat. People with celiac disease often experience an improvement in their symptoms simply by eliminating all wheat and wheat products from their diet. Screening for celiac disease is performed using a blood test, or alternatively, the gold standard would be to perform a biopsy of the lining of the small intestine.

Colonoscopy

A standard of practice is that all people fifty years old or older have a colonoscopy to check for possible colon cancer and to screen for polyps in an effort to prevent colon cancer. Any patient older than the age of fifty with changes in bowel habits should be considered for colonoscopy. This is important since the incidence of colon cancer increases with age. In patients younger than fifty, colonoscopy can rule out diseases such as Crohn's disease or ulcerative colitis (both conditions of inflammation in the intestine or colon), which can have symptoms that mimic IBS. Colonoscopy for patients younger than fifty years old should be considered on a case-by-case basis.

Thyroid Testing

I also ask my patients to have their thyroid levels tested to ensure that their thyroid function is normal. Elevated or reduced thyroid levels can often contribute to diarrhea or constipation, respectively.

All of the above are tests that my colleagues and I insist that all of our IBS patients undergo because we want to make sure that their health maintenance is properly addressed. If you are experiencing IBS-like symptoms, you should have your physician consider these or similar tests as well.

Once I have eliminated all other potential factors that can cause

RECOMMENDED TESTS	WARNING SIGNS
	(That This May Not Be IBS)
1. A good history and physical (nothing can replace this)	1. Blood in stool
2. Complete blood count (CBC)	2. Constant diarrhea (The bowel habits in IBS usually fluctuate.)
3. Erythrocyte sedimentation rate (ESR)	
4. Celiac blood testing	3. Fever
5. Stool studies for blood, and culture for pathogenic bacteria and parasites	4. Diarrhea at night
	5. Weight loss
	6. Age over fifty years (consider colonoscopy)
6. Endoscopic examination (on a case-by-case basis)	7. Vomiting

IBS-like symptoms, I have our patients take the breath test that was explained in Chapter 5. Usually, they will see me later on the same day the breath test is performed, so that I can go over the results with them and outline an appropriate course of treatment. If the breath test indicates bacterial overgrowth, the next step is to have them begin the Cedars-Sinai protocol for IBS.

THE PROTOCOL

Based on the findings of the breath test, I am able to determine whether or not my patients have bacterial overgrowth. If they test positive for bacterial overgrowth, I place them on a course of antibiotic treatment for an initial ten-day period. The use of antibiotics can eradicate bacterial overgrowth, regardless of whether patients test positive for methane gas, in which case their IBS symptoms are most probably constipation predominant, or for hydrogen gas, in which case their IBS symptoms can vary.

There are two antibiotics that I recommend for treating the bacterial overgrowth associated with IBS. The first drug, which is the one I most commonly prescribe, is called rifaximin (trade name Xifaxan), which is manufactured by Salix, a pharmaceutical company that is actively researching effective ways of treating IBS. I might also prescribe neomycin.

I recommend rifaximin and neomycin for two reasons. The first reason is because both drugs have been shown to be effective for eradicating bacterial overgrowth. The second reason, which helps explain why they are so useful in treating intestinal bacterial overgrowth, is because only very small amounts of these drugs are absorbed by the bloodstream. In the case of rifaximin, 99.6 percent of it stays in the gastrointestinal tract, while approximately 95 percent of neomycin does the same. This is an important point. Unlike other, more absorbable antibiotics, instead of being dispersed through the bloodstream to other areas of the body, rifaximin and neomycin remain inside the gastrointestinal tract, making them more effective. In addition, the non-absorbability of both rifaximin and neomycin makes them far less likely to cause side effects in other parts of the body.

In both drugs, there are minimal side effects. Therefore, for example, female patients are far less likely to develop vaginal yeast infections, and neither drug is likely to affect bacteria in other areas of the body, thereby avoiding the problem of bacterial resistance, which is a major reason that so many other drugs, over time, lose their effectiveness. The safety and effectiveness of both rifaximin and neomycin makes them ideal choices for treating intestinal bacterial overgrowth.

This is especially the case with rifaximin, as shown by a study that my colleagues and I conducted regarding its effectiveness for treating IBS. In the study, which involved eighty-seven patients, there were two remarkable findings. First, the study demonstrated that the patients' IBS symptoms significantly decreased after a single ten-day course of rifaximin. More important, the symptom improvement lasted for two months after treatment. This is the first treatment for IBS that does not require continuous administration of drug to be effective, and this provides proof that we are treating a cause of IBS.

One issue about rifaximin is that it is FDA approved for traveler's diarrhea but not for IBS. This can be a problem for insurance coverage of the drug. Hopefully, once the insurance carriers realize that this is a single ten-day course rather than continuous therapy (not to mention fewer healthcare provider visits for IBS patients), they will be more apt to cover the prescriptions.

Once the ten-day course of antibiotic treatment ends, I then administer a follow-up breath test for my patients, which is usually scheduled within five days after they have taken their final dose of the antibiotic. Before proceeding to the next phase of the protocol, the follow-up breath test has to be negative, meaning that the levels of methane and/or hydrogen gas have returned to normal.

If the follow-up breath test is negative, patients should be free or nearly free of their symptoms. However, if the follow-up breath test shows incomplete eradication of the bacteria, the patient is likely to have only partial symptom relief.

In cases where the patient reports a 90 to 95 percent improvement in their symptoms, the treatment can be considered a success, and there is no need to prescribe a further course of antibiotics, regardless of the breath test results. But in cases where the improvement is only 60 to 70 percent and breath test improvement is partial, I will discuss with patients the possibility that another course of antibiotic treatment will result in further improvements. If they agree, I will prescribe a combination of rifaximin with neomycin. In such cases, their initial improvements usually become even more pronounced. As a word of caution, if the breath test becomes normal after the antibiotic treatment but there is no improvement in symptoms (or only a slight improvement), one should consider another diagnosis. For example, it is common for patients with Crohn's disease to have bacterial overgrowth because this condition can cause partial blockage of the small intestine and decrease drainage. In addition, celiac disease has even been associated with bacterial overgrowth.

Once the bacterial overgrowth has been eradicated to a satisfactory degree, the next step of the Cedars-Sinai protocol for IBS involves restoring the normal function of the cleansing waves of the small intestine. This is crucial because proper function of the cleansing waves minimizes the likelihood of future episodes of bacterial overgrowth. My colleagues and I accomplish this by having our IBS patients take either erythromycin, in a dose of 50 milligrams, or Zelnorm, in a dosage range of 2 to 6 milligrams, at bedtime.

Both of these products have been shown to enhance small bowel cleansing waves. I prescribe these drugs to be taken at bedtime, because while the patient is not eating, the body is producing the most cleansing-wave activity. Typically, patients take these drugs for a three-month period, following the eradication of bacterial overgrowth. They then return to see me so that I can discuss with them their options for going forward.

Basically, at three months, patients have two options. They can either stop taking their prescribed medication (erythromycin or Zelnorm), or they can continue taking it because they find that they are continuing to feel much better and experiencing few if any symptoms. My preference is that they eventually stop taking the drugs, because I am not in favor of the indefinite use of medications. My goal as a physician is to help my patients return to a state of normal health and then be free to get on with their lives without the need for medications. However, if patients choose to stop the preventive therapy, I will point out that the possibility exists that they may later experience a recurrence of their bacterial overgrowth. In that case, the solution is simple: the patient will simply need to begin the protocol again. Those patients who, for whatever reason, are unable to regain normal cleansing-wave activity without the use of medication may then need to stay on erythromycin or Zelnorm indefinitely.

In some instances, at three months, patients express their satisfaction with the results of the protocol and choose to continue taking erythromycin or Zelnorm beyond the three-month period because they feel well and don't want to risk a return of their IBS symptoms. These patients return for follow-up every three to six months so that I can be sure their progress is being maintained and that the drugs are not causing any side effects.

Overall, both erythromycin and Zelnorm are very safe at the dosage levels that we are prescribing. It should be mentioned, however, that erythromycin may affect the heart's electrical cycle, but evidence suggests this risk is usually associated with much higher doses (up to 2,000 milligrams per day), not with the 50-milligram dose that is shown to improve gut movement. Still, because of this potential side effect, patients who elect to take erythromycin should do so only under a physician's ongoing supervision, especially if they are already at risk for developing cardiovascular disease.

Another cautionary note concerns women in their potential childbearing years. During the maintenance phase of the protocol, patients may decide to become pregnant. I let my female patients know before we begin the preventive maintenance phase that they are to let me know if they are considering pregnancy. If they are, then I will have them stop taking erythromycin or Zelnorm. Although Zelnorm and erythromycin taken during pregnancy are not associated with risks, I prefer to be overly cautious. Aside from these factors, I find the preventive maintenance phase of the protocol using erythromycin or Zelnorm to be safe even when it is followed indefinitely, so long as it is undertaken with a physician's supervision.

VIVONEX

In cases of bacterial overgrowth that remains resistant even after one or more ten-day antibiotic treatments using rifaximin or neomycin, I will often recommend that patients follow a two-week diet in which they drink only water and replace all three of their daily meals with Vivonex.

Vivonex is an elemental food formula that contains all of a person's recommended daily allowances for the vitamins, minerals, essential fatty acids, and other nutrients that the body requires to properly function. Vivonex consists of completely predigested proteins, fats, and carbohydrates. Instead of proteins, it contains amino acids, which are the building blocks of protein. It also contains the fatty acids that the body needs, as well as carbohydrate in the form of glucose, a simple sugar that is so readily absorbed by humans that there is little left for the gut bacteria to feed on.

Vivonex, which is manufactured by Novartis Nutrition, is manufactured in such a way that people can live on it indefinitely if they had to. Because it is predigested, it is extremely gentle and easy for the gastrointestinal tract to absorb. All of the ingredients in Vivonex get absorbed within about the first two feet of the gastrointestinal tract, often well before reaching the areas where bacterial overgrowth would usually occur. Research conducted since the 1970s has shown that a diet consisting exclusively of Vivonex and water can significantly reduce overall bacterial overload. In tests conducted by my colleagues and me involving over one hundred IBS patients, bacterial overgrowth was eradicated in more than 80 percent of all cases after the Vivonex diet was followed for two weeks, making it one of the most effective ways for addressing bacterial overgrowth. In fact, we have now treated more than 800 patients with IBS/bacterial overgrowth this way with this rate of success.

During the time that patients are following the Vivonex diet, no antibiotics are administered. In fact, taking antibiotics during this two-week period is generally counterproductive. The reason for this is that antibiotics work only on bacteria that are replicating or reproducing.

Because of how effective Vivonex is at starving bacteria, the bacteria go into a hibernating, nonreplicating mode. Hibernating bacteria, in general, are not as susceptible to antibiotics.

Although Vivonex is available over the counter, without the need for a physician's prescription, I do not recommend that IBS patients attempt this diet without first informing their doctors. In addition, it is important that Vivonex be consumed in sufficient quantities each day so that the patient's caloric needs are met; otherwise, there is the risk of unwanted weight loss. Moreover, I don't recommend this diet for patients with diabetes or kidney disease, and especially not for patients who are receiving dialysis, without their doctors' approval.

Beyond those cautions, my colleagues and I have found Vivonex to be one of the most effective methods for eradicating bacterial overgrowth. (Vivonex is discussed in further detail in Chapter 7.)

DIETARY DO'S AND DON'TS

The key dietary strategy, especially during the maintenance phase of the Cedars-Sinai protocol for IBS, which is focused on eradicating bacterial overgrowth, is to avoid eating foods upon which bacteria thrive. For the most part, this means eliminating hard-to-digest sugars (with the exception of glucose, which is readily absorbed within the first two feet of the gastrointestinal tract), as sugar is the most important nutrient for bacteria, along with a small degree of hydration (water), in order to thrive and reproduce.

The diet that I devised and recommend is therefore a low-carbohydrate diet that also limits lactose, a simple sugar found in milk and other dairy products.

Many IBS patients, as well as a large portion of the population in general, are considered to be lactose intolerant, meaning that they have difficulty digesting lactose. My colleagues and I showed in a study that the symptoms of lactose intolerance are, in fact, caused by the bacteria in the small intestine feeding on lactose to cause bloating and other problems. Lactose must go through the entire fifteen feet of the small intestine before the body can digest and assimilate it, making it an ideal simple sugar for bacteria in the distant parts of the small bowel to feed upon. In most cases, however, once the bacteria is eradicated, patients find that they can then consume lactose-containing foods with far fewer, if any, symptoms because the bacteria are no longer there to interact with the lactose. However, continuing to eat lactose-containing foods may encourage the bacteria to return. Drinking Lactaid milk (in which the lactose is predigested) is encouraged.

Sugar substitutes, or artificial sweeteners like Splenda, are also advised against. Such products are advertised as being low- or zero-calorie alternatives to sugar. This is because they are sugars that humans are unable to digest. These sugars are eaten but not absorbed, so the bacteria of the gut feed on it and can continue to replicate. Essentially, when it comes to substitutes for sugar like sucralose or sorbitol, it's "zero calories for you, 100 percent calories for your gut bacteria" and is the common reason for bloating associated with chewing sugar-free gum.

Dietary Guidelines for Helping to Eradicate Bacteria Overgrowth and Prevent Its Return

Traditionally, the diet for people with IBS was one that encourages the consumption of high-fiber foods along with plenty of fluids to increase bowel motility and to relieve constipation. In addition, patients were often advised to eat five to six smaller meals during the day, instead of the normal, larger three meals that most people commonly eat. Unfortunately, both of these measures—high-fiber diets and more frequent meals—were counterproductive for most patients with IBS.

The problem with fiber is that it is comprised of carbohydrate chains that humans can't digest. The undigested fiber supplements make their way down to the colon, where the bacteria ferment it, producing bloating. Therefore, I recommend a diet that contains only modest amounts of fiber found naturally in fruits and vegetables, in place of fiber supplements intended as stool-bulking agents. I think you're getting the idea: don't eat food that leaves much behind.

Eating more than three meals a day also causes problems for people with IBS. The reason for this is that the cleansing-wave mechanism that rids the small intestine of food byproducts, waste, and bacteria can only occur when you're not eating. The more meals that you have per day—and this includes snacks between meals—the less time your body has to produce appropriate cleansing waves, making it easier for the bacteria in the small intestine to maintain their colonization.

The dietary approach that I recommend to my IBS patients is to eat foods that are easily digested, so that most of the nutrients can be absorbed higher up in the intestine, away from bacteria. In this case, less "residue" is left over at the distal, or "bottom" end. Your diet should contain some fiber for bulk and proper stool formation, but not too much, and it should be primarily composed of foods that are easily absorbed.

Foods that are *not* well absorbed should be minimized or eliminated from the diet altogether, because they end up being a good fuel source for the bacteria residing near the "bottom" of the small intestine.

Adequate fluid intake throughout the day is also important. If your diet does not include enough water, it becomes more difficult for your body to have proper bowel motility. Without healthy bowel movement, the buildup of bacteria within the gastrointestinal tract becomes more likely.

Finally, as I mentioned, it is important that you limit your food intake to three meals per day, eating nothing in between. This means that you allow three to five hours between each meal, and avoid snacks and drinks (other than water) during that time, so that the small intestine's cleansing-wave function can take place. For those patients who are most prone to bacterial overgrowth, the cleansing-wave function may not be very efficient. This is why it is particularly important that you give the small intestine a break from food for three to five hours between meals to allow the cleansing function a chance to rid the intestine of food residue and bacteria.

What follows are ten guidelines on how to eat in order to most effectively reduce and prevent bacterial overgrowth. These guidelines should also be followed after you complete the IBS protocol and have eradicated bacterial overgrowth, so that you have the best chance of minimizing its return.

1. Try to avoid the following sweeteners:
   - Corn syrup (fructose)
   - Mannitol
   - Sorbitol
   - Sucralose (Splenda)
   - Lactose
   - Lactulose

The biggest culprit is sugar-free gum, which most often contains sorbitol (a sugar that humans cannot digest). On the other hand, glucose, sucrose (table sugar), and aspartame (Equal or Nutrasweet) are acceptable. You should also limit foods and food products sweetened with fruit juice, which contains fructose. This is hard because so many food products are sweetened with fructose. Try to limit your sugar intake to no more than 40 grams per day, and ideally much less. Reading food labels can help you achieve your goal.

2. Limit or eliminate the following "high-residue" foods. These foods are difficult to digest and leave residue in the small intestine:

   - Beans (kidney beans, garbanzo beans, pinto beans, etc.)
   - Lentils
   - Peas (including split-pea soup)
   - Soy products (tofu, soymilk)
   - Yogurt, milk, and cheese (100-percent Lactaid milk is acceptable as a milk substitute.)

3. Drink eight cups of water a day. A good guideline is to drink two cups of water with each of your three meals, then one cup between breakfast and lunch, and one cup between lunch and dinner.

4. Beef, fish, poultry, and eggs are acceptable foods, and are also good sources of protein. You do not need to limit these foods throughout the day. However, be sure to only eat portions that are appropriate for your body size. Most people require only about 4–8 ounces of meat products per day.

5. Potatoes, pasta, rice, bread, and cereals are also acceptable. It's all right to include some of these foods at each meal. They contain carbohydrates that are well absorbed high up in the small intestine, serving as fuel for your body, not for the bacteria. A good rule of thumb is to eat no more than a half cup to one cup of these carbohydrate foods at each meal. Believe it or not, white bread is best in this circumstance. Try to keep multigrain breads to a minimum. If whole-grain breads are desired, oat and wheat fibers are better choices. Also avoid wild rice.

6. Fruits should be eaten in moderation—two servings per day. Fruits contain fructose, which again is difficult to digest. Choose fresh, not dried fruit. Dried fruits concentrate the fructose into a smaller package and it allows for more fructose ingestion because more is eaten.

7. Fresh, nonstarchy vegetables should also be part of your daily food intake. Cooked or lightly steamed vegetables are preferable to raw

vegetables, because they are easier to digest and absorb. Avoid large salads full of raw vegetables, as this can lead to too much residue. You can incorporate small amounts of salad, but do not eat raw vegetables exclusively as they are hard to digest. A good rule of thumb is to have three to five cups of cooked vegetables per day.

8. Dairy products are best avoided because of the lactose they contain. In addition, do not substitute with soymilk, as soy products contain nonabsorbable oligosaccharides, a class of carbohydrate that can contribute to bloating. Try almond or rice milk instead. Another great alternative is Lactaid milk, because all of the lactose is predigested.

9. Coffee, tea, and soda should be consumed only in moderate amounts. Out of these three types of beverages, tea is probably the most healthful choice. Coffee is also acceptable as long as you limit your intake to one or two cups per day. Sodas, on the other hand, are not a healthy choice. Non-diet sodas may contain corn syrup and other types of sugar. Diet sodas are now starting to contain sucralose (Splenda), another fuel source for bacteria. These types of soda should be avoided altogether. Diet sodas containing Nutrasweet may be consumed in moderation. When you are thirsty, however, the best option is to have pure, filtered water. Water flavored with lemon or lime juice is also a good alternative.

10. Finally, make sure you eat a balanced diet and that your meals contain sufficient calories so that you are able to maintain your body weight. In addition, incorporate moderate exercise into your weekly routine at least every other day, as regular physical activity helps to maintain regular bowel movements.

A FIVE-DAY MENU PLAN

The following five-day menu plan can help to reduce symptoms of IBS that are caused by bacterial overgrowth, because it limits your intake of the sugars and simple carbohydrates that bacteria consume. After the five days are over, you can repeat the diet, starting over with the food plan for Day One, or you can improvise, following the dietary guidelines described earlier.

DAY ONE

Breakfast
Scrambled eggs
1 piece white-bread toast
with margarine
Coffee or herbal tea
1–2 cups of water

Mid-Day
1 cup of water

Lunch
Tuna-fish sandwich
on lightly toasted white bread
1 cup of vegetable soup
Coffee or herbal tea
1–2 cups of water

Mid-Afternoon
1 cup of water

Dinner
Baked chicken
1 baked potato with chives and/or margarine
1 serving of steamed asparagus
2 cups of water
Cluster of grapes for dessert

Mid-Evening
1 cup of water

DAY TWO

Breakfast

1 bowl of puffed-rice cereal
with Lactaid milk

Coffee or herbal tea

1–2 cups of water

Mid-Day

1 cup of water

Lunch

Broiled chicken

Small salad

Coffee or herbal tea

1–2 cups of water

Mid-Afternoon

1 cup of water

Dinner

Steak

Rice topped with medley
of steamed vegetables
(carrots, zucchini, and squash)

2 cups of water

Mid-Evening

1 cup of water

DAY THREE

Breakfast

Mushroom omelette (no cheese)

1 piece white-bread toast with margarine

Coffee or herbal tea

1–2 cups of water

Mid-Day

1 cup of water

Lunch

Turkey burger on sesame-seed
white-bread bun

1 cup of tomato soup

Coffee or herbal tea

1–2 cups of water

Mid-Afternoon

1 cup of water

Dinner

Baked halibut

Roasted portabello mushrooms

Small salad

2 cups of water

Mid-Evening

1 cup of water

DAY FOUR

Breakfast
1 cup of cream of wheat
(with Lactaid, almond, or rice milk)
Coffee or herbal tea
2 cups of water

Mid-Day
1 cup of water

Lunch
Tomato basil linguini
1 small white-bread roll
Roasted beets
Diet soda (with aspartame)
Coffee or herbal tea
1–2 cups of water

Mid-Afternoon
1 cup of water

Dinner
Rosemary leg of lamb
Sautéed vegetables
Small serving of garlic mashed potatoes
2 cups of water

Mid-Evening
1 cup of water

DAY FIVE

Breakfast
Sausage and eggs
1 piece white-bread toast with margarine
Coffee or herbal tea
1–2 cups of water

Mid-Day
1 cup of water

Lunch
Soup and small salad
Coffee or herbal tea
1–2 cups of water

Mid-Afternoon
1 cup of water

Dinner
Broiled salmon with lemon
Cooked carrots
1 cup of rice or 1 baked potato
2 cups of water

Mid-Evening
1 cup of water

CASE HISTORY

My colleagues and I have successfully helped innumerable IBS patients take control of their symptoms to regain a good quality of life, including many patients whose symptoms were extremely severe and seemingly intractable. One such patient was Marjorie Pendergraft, who suffered with severe and debilitating symptoms of IBS for many years before she came to me. Her successful experience with the Cedars-Sinai protocol, which she recounts below, illustrates how effective it is for treating IBS.

> I don't think I ever had normal bowel habits until I met Dr. Pimentel. I had always had some difficulty with my bowels. I had had all sorts of tests, but they couldn't find anything wrong. Then I began to get a lot worse. My symptoms became acute, and for eleven years I suffered with stomach trouble, indigestion, and nearly constant diarrhea. My diarrhea got to the point where I was afraid to go out of the house until I had made five or six trips to the bathroom in the mornings and was cleared out. This affected my life a great deal, and along with it came this tremendous feeling of malaise that was eventually diagnosed as chronic fatigue syndrome. Now, I don't know what chronic fatigue syndrome is, and I don't know that anybody does. But I had lots of strange symptoms and aches and just a general sense of not feeling well.
>
> Finally, things reached a point to where it was beyond my ability to hold a job. I was on disability for about a year. My symptoms were acute more often than not, and I just didn't feel good. In addition to the diarrhea, I usually experienced bloating and a sense of fullness, and I would get a rash and other allergic reactions to certain foods, especially anything that was acidic. At times I was also emotionally despondent. Since I was operating on the assumption that my symptoms were due to chronic fatigue syndrome, since that was what my doctor had told me, I didn't know anything about IBS. When I read that the Director of the National Institutes of Health said that chronic fatigue is nothing but clinical depression, my response, which I've used ever since then with skeptics, is that if you had it, you would not call it clinical depression.

When I went to my doctor, I was given low dosage antidepressants because my doctor said that it very often helped the
chronic fatigue. I ended up being prescribed a whole bunch of
different antidepressants. Some had such bad side effects that I
couldn't even get out of bed. I was an absolute a zombie, and
I immediately stopped taking them. I would try others for a
while, but they just didn't help.

I continued to undergo tests to rule out anything serious,
and the doctors kept telling me that everything looked just fine.
I was very frustrated by this. My closest friend, who was an
occupational therapist, told me, "Marge, you shouldn't be cross;
the findings are good news. They've ruled out all of the things
that could kill you." I replied that I was cross and disgusted
because I still didn't have any answers about what was making
me feel so terrible.

The only times I seemed to experience any relief was whenever I received a course of antibiotics. I had an impacted tooth,
for instance, and received antibiotics, and after that I felt better
for a while. At that time I had no idea there could be a connection between the antibiotics and my symptoms. But now I can
see that the antibiotics helped a good deal with the situation I
now know to call "bacterial overgrowth."

Other than those few times, I continued to suffer, until I
finally learned about Dr. Pimentel's work. One of my friends
suggested I speak with her cousin, whose symptoms sounded
a lot like mine. The woman described everything she had gone
through, and then told me about the work that they were doing
at Cedars-Sinai Medical Center. What she told me about bacterial overgrowth was the first description I had ever heard that
I could connect with. So I went to Cedars-Sinai, and I had all of
the tests in the motility unit. That's when I met Dr. Pimentel. I
told him, "This is the first time I have ever heard anything
about my condition that makes perfect sense to me. It feels like
my body's been poisoning itself with these bacteria proliferat-
ing inside of me and sending all these toxins throughout my
system."

Dr. Pimentel replied that the bacterial overgrowth was what
he and his colleagues believed was causing people like me to

have symptoms. But he also scheduled me for a colonoscopy to rule out anything else. I had that, and the results were negative. Then I had the breath test, which was very simple and comfortable to do, and it indicated that I had bacterial overgrowth, just as we suspected. Dr. Pimentel gave me a prescription for neomycin and I began to take it each day.

For the first five days, I thought it wasn't working. In fact, my symptoms were getting worse. Then, on the sixth day, when I woke up in the morning, for the first time I felt comfortable inside my skin. Even the bed felt softer and more comfortable than it had for a long, long time. I told my husband, "I feel good! I feel better than I have felt in years!"

When I returned for my follow-up with Dr. Pimentel, I explained that I didn't think the neomycin was working at first because I'd started feeling worse, not better. He told me that he thought the reason for my initial discomfort was because all of the bacteria were "giving up the ghost and releasing more toxins," but once that passed I got better. "Oh, boy," I replied. "Did I ever!" It was a dramatic improvement. It was like somebody had flipped a switch.

That was seven years ago. Since then, my entire life has been renewed. I can do practically anything now, and it's just miraculous. Right after I finished my treatment, I told Dr. Pimentel that I felt twenty years younger, and I still do. Since that time, my husband and I moved up to Seattle from Los Angeles, and recently we have been remodeling our home, tearing down walls, painting all of the rooms, and I'm just having a ball. I couldn't have done that before!

Not only are my IBS symptoms much, much better, but I also have tremendous amounts of energy and I can go for very long periods of time without experiencing problems. If my symptoms flare up again, as they do on occasion, I go back to Dr. Pimentel for another round of antibiotics. Now he prescribes neomycin in combination with rifaximin, and that works even better. I'm so grateful that he and his colleagues have been doing this research. Since I've found out about him, I've had people call me with their own IBS symptoms and I've referred them all to Dr. Pimentel because his approach really works!

CONCLUSION

Now that you've read this far, you know not only what causes most cases of IBS, but also how to treat it most effectively. As Marjorie's story shows, the Cedars-Sinai protocol for IBS is often the only thing that has enabled patients to regain control of their lives and become free of their symptoms. It is highly effective for the vast majority of IBS patients who consult with my colleagues and me. Some patients, however, are interested in combining the protocol with other alternative healing approaches. In the next chapter, I provide information about which of those therapies have value as an adjunctive aid to the Cedars-Sinai protocol for IBS, and which of them are of little value.

SUMMARY OF THE CEDARS-SINAI PROTOCOL FOR IBS

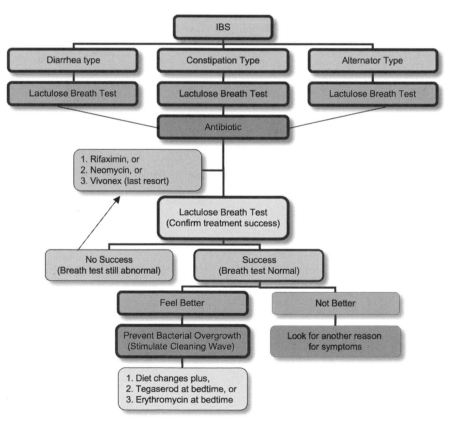

CHAPTER 7

The Best of Both Worlds:
Enhancing Your Results
With Alternative Therapies

By now you understand our strategy for treating IBS based on the presence of bacterial overgrowth as discussed in Chapter 6. However, there are a number of "alternative" therapies that some people with IBS find useful for helping to manage their symptoms. This chapter is devoted to examining the most common of these alternatives and providing you with a better understanding of why they may or may not be useful. I will also try to place their benefits in the context of the bacterial theory where appropriate. Bear in mind that some of these alternatives do not reduce bacterial overgrowth to any significant degree. For some people, however, these techniques can help to alleviate symptoms associated with IBS.

PROBIOTICS

As I discussed in Chapter 4, probiotics are commonly referred to as "good" bacteria and probiotic supplements are often used as a means of increasing the supply of "good" bacteria in the gastrointestinal tract, while holding "bad" bacteria in check. Actually, when it comes to the gastrointestinal tract, the concept of "good" bacteria is a misnomer. As I mentioned in Chapter 4, very few, if any, of the approximately 400 different strains of bacteria in the gastrointestinal are in fact "bad" or "good." Rather, they simply represent the various strains of bacteria that are normally found in the colon (or large intestine). It is when these strains of bacteria leave the areas of the gastrointestinal tract in which they properly belong that problems can occur.

Our understanding of the role bacteria play in the gastrointestinal tract, as well as the degree to which their various populations are within normal limits, is at present incomplete. In fact, we are only able to culture 20 percent of the gut bacteria because we do not understand how to grow the remaining 80 percent. This keeps us from finding out which bacteria or combinations may be helpful or harmful. For this reason, researchers are now conducting genetic studies on all of the microorganisms that occur in the gastrointestinal tract in an attempt to determine the cellular "fingerprint" of the various strains of bacteria as a means of figuring out which strains are most likely to predominate in the normal gut. This type of research could go a long way toward helping us understand how all of the strains of bacteria in the gastrointestinal tract contribute to both health and disease.

At present, people with IBS are all too often advised to have a stool sample cultured to see whether or not they have adequate amounts of certain "good" bacteria, such as lactobacillus (especially the strains *L. acidophilus* and *L. bulgaricus*) or bifidobacteria. If the levels of these types of bacteria are found to be low, it is often recommended that they be replenished via supplementation so that the IBS patient will feel better. This approach is based on data suggesting that IBS subjects have lower lactobacillus numbers in their stool especially if they have diarrhea-predominant IBS. We now know that probiotic supplementation overall has shown little long-term benefit for IBS patients.

A number of controlled studies showed limited benefits. In one study, IBS patients were given a probiotic product called VSL #3. Compared with patients in the control group, the patients who took the product showed modest improvement in bloating. In another study, IBS patients were given isolated strains of bifidobacteria (*B. infantis*) or an isolated strain of lactobacillus (*L. salivarius*). The benefits produced by the lactobacillus were statistically nonexistent, while the patients given bifidobacteria showed some reduction of their IBS symptoms as long as they continued taking the supplement.

In still another double-blind study, involving fifty patients with IBS, test subjects received *L. plantarum* LP0 1 (another lactobacillus strain) and *B. breve* BR0 (a type of bifidobacteria) or placebo powder for a period of twenty-eight days. After twenty-eight days, 49 percent of the probiotic group showed improvements in their abdominal pain, compared with 29 percent of the placebo group.

While a reduction in IBS symptoms is certainly a good outcome, it is not the same as the elimination of IBS itself. According to current scientific study, probiotics have not been found to eliminate IBS.

Another problem with probiotic supplementation is that the cleansing waves in the small intestines of IBS patients are inadequate. It's possible that a person with diminished cleansing-wave capacity who takes probiotic supplements could find his or her situation even worse as the probiotics accumulate in the small intestine, where they don't belong.

On the other hand, an animal study conducted by European researchers has shown that certain bifidobacteria and lactobacillus may stimulate the cleansing-wave mechanism. In the study, animals were purposely bred so that they lacked any bacteria (germ free). When they were given either bifidobacteria or lactobacillus, a stimulation of cleansing-wave activity was observed. However, the conclusions from this study may not apply to us because our bodies contain a multitude of bacterial strains.

In concluding this discussion of probiotics, I want to point out that certain strains of "good" bacteria may provide some relief of the severity of IBS symptoms. At this stage in our understanding of probiotics, as well as gastrointestinal bacteria in general, it remains too early to know the best approach for using probiotics. Future studies may show that they do indeed have a place in the overall treatment for IBS. Thus far, they only appear to provide symptom relief, and not provide a comprehensive solution for IBS such as that provided by our protocol.

DIET

Diet certainly has a place when it comes to treating IBS. Eating healthily and wisely, for example, is a good way of preventing food poisoning, which is often a "trigger event" for IBS symptoms. It also goes without saying that we should do our best to eat foods that are free of chemical additives and preservatives as much as possible, and to avoid the processed and "junk" fast foods that are unfortunately a major part of the American diet. As we discussed earlier, people withIBS should also reduce the intake of foods and drinks that contain sugars and other simple carbohydrates, the prime nutrients for bacteria.

To see for yourself how powerfully sugar attracts and nourishes bacteria, try this simple experiment. Pour equal amounts of water into two clear glasses. Add some sugar to one of the glasses, and then set both glasses on a countertop overnight. Next morning, the glass without sugar will still be clear, while the glass with sugar will be cloudy due to bacteria that found their way into the water to feed on the sugar. The longer the glass with sugar is set out, the cloudier it will become as the bacteria grow and multiply.

A similar process occurs in the body when sugars and other simple carbohydrates are regularly made available for bacteria. People with IBS who regularly eat foods containing sugars and other simple carbohydrates (such as refined flour, another common staple ingredient in fast and processed foods) are actually making their IBS symptoms worse.

The key here is not that all sugars are bad, but that the less digestible sugars are available in larger amounts for fermentation by small bowel bacteria. Most of the sugars found in so many of today's processed foods are not easy for the body to digest. As a result, these sugars are able to travel through much of the full length of the small bowel, reaching areas where bacteria can feast upon them. Lactose, a milk sugar, falls into this category. The lactose in one glass of milk requires nearly the entire length of the gastrointestinal tract in order to be absorbed by the body because there is not enough lactase, the enzyme that breaks down lactose, in the small intestine. In addition, lactose intolerance increases with age, making it increasingly difficult for adults to properly digest. So, even something as seemingly innocuous as a glass of milk can worsen bacterial overgrowth.

By the time they see a doctor, most IBS patients have already discovered that milk or other dairy products make their symptoms worse and have already omitted them from their diets. Although avoiding milk products does not eliminate IBS symptoms, patients complain that the milk products aggravate their symptoms. Other non-digestible sugars that I advise my IBS patients to avoid or reduce include fructose (corn syrup), which is nearly ubiquitous in today's commercial food products; maltose; maltitol; sucralose (Splenda); sorbitol; and lactulose. Sugar substitutes such as sorbitol and sucralose are two of the worst. Both are non-digestible carbohydrates that are known to cause or exacerbate bloating and gas, and may alter bowel function.

Because sugars and other carbohydrates can exacerbate IBS symptoms, many IBS patients are turning to low-carbohydrate diets such as the South Beach Diet and, especially, the Atkins Diet. I've been told by many of my IBS patients, and have confirmed this in my clinic, that after they adopt such diets, they begin to notice a decrease in their severity of their symptoms. They feel less bloated, have less gas, and less pain in their stomachs. But as soon as they resume eating carbohydrates, their symptoms soon become as bad as or worse than before.

I caution my patients about staying on the Atkins Diet for long periods of time, because it overemphasizes protein-rich foods, and I doubt that even Dr. Atkins expected that people would follow the extreme early stage of his diet indefinitely. In the short term, the Atkins and similar diets can help alleviate IBS symptoms. As a healthier alternative, I recommend that IBS patients make it a habit to eliminate or at least severely restrict their intake of the non-digestible forms of sugars and other simple carbohydrates mentioned above, focusing instead on (ideally organic) fresh and non-starchy vegetables, fish, poultry, and in moderation red meat, while also avoiding sodas and fruit juices (especially commercial brands), all of which are high in sugar content. This deprives the bacteria of their primary food sources, so they cannot grow and multiply.

Glucose: The Healthy Sugar

While other forms of sugar can hurt your health, there is one form of sugar that is not only good for you, but is also essential for the proper function of your body. That sugar is glucose.

Glucose is the most important carbohydrate for your body's metabolism. All of the cells and tissues, especially of the brain and nervous system, use glucose to produce energy. In addition, unlike other sugars, glucose does not contribute to the proliferation of bacteria in the gastrointestinal tract because it gets absorbed in the body too quickly, never reaching the small intestine, where bacteria overgrowth typically occurs.

The Elemental Diet

For IBS patients with severe bacterial overgrowth, adopting what I call an "elemental diet" for a few weeks can often significantly improve IBS symptoms, as well as eradicate bacterial overgrowth. The diet involves abstaining from all solid food for two weeks, and instead consuming the product Vivonex and drinking only water.

Vivonex is available over the counter at most local drugstores. This dietary approach is an "elemental diet" because Vivonex consists of the elemental building blocks for each of the major food categories—proteins, carbohydrates, and fats.

Instead of proteins, it contains amino acids; instead of complex fats, it contains fatty acids; and instead of carbohydrate chains, it contains glucose. As long as enough Vivonex is consumed to ensure proper caloric intake, it provides everything that the human body needs. Moreover, because the constituents of each food group are already broken down, the product is extremely easy for the body to absorb.

My colleagues and I published a study in *Digestive Diseases and Sciences* in 2003, in which we placed approximately one hundred IBS patients on Vivonex for two weeks. Within that period, more than 80 percent of them had their bacterial overgrowth completely eradicated, making the elemental diet one of the most effective approaches for dealing with IBS.

The challenge is getting patients to stay on the diet, since it is only natural that they might begin to crave some other type of food during the two-week period. In addition, some people balk at the cost of Vivonex—a two-week supply retails for approximately $450. And because Vivonex is an over-the-counter nutritional supplement, most insurance companies won't cover the expense. But as I tell my patients, the cost of Vivonex is insignificant compared with the benefits they will achieve if they follow the diet for two weeks as recommended—not to mention the money they will save on other treatments that do little to nothing to relieve their symptoms of IBS. By far, the elemental diet is the most effective self-care approach for IBS because it nourishes the body while at the same time it provides no nourishment for the bacteria that cause IBS. For best results, however, I recommend that the elemental diet be conducted under the supervision of a physician.

PEPPERMINT CAPSULES

To help relieve the cramping so often associated with IBS, enteric-coated peppermint capsules can sometimes be helpful. Peppermint has been shown to be a calcium channel blocker of muscle. Calcium channel blockers get their name because of their ability to block calcium fluctuations in the muscle cells, thereby causing muscles to relax.

Enteric-coated peppermint capsules have been shown in a scientific meta-analysis (an analysis of numerous studies) to provide some degree of benefit for IBS. In many cases, the benefits were modest, yet nonetheless real and statistically significant, in terms of reducing cramping within the gastrointestinal tract. Based on its ability to act as a calcium channel blocker, researchers presume these benefits are due to the peppermint's ability to relax the muscles of the stomach, small intestine, and colon. As a result, these muscles are less likely to contract against gases, and therefore the sensations of high pressure in the abdomen will usually be less painful. In addition, there have been case reports that indicate peppermint may also have some degree of effectiveness as an antibacterial agent, so the possibility exists that enteric-coated peppermint might also help arrest bacterial overgrowth.

To achieve the above benefits, the peppermint needs to be enteric-coated to protect it from being broken down and digested prior to reaching those areas of the gastrointestinal tract. Other forms of peppermint, such as peppermint tea, may not give the same benefits because they are broken down by the time they reach the esophagus and stomach. Enteric-coated peppermint should be available at your local health food store.

PANCREATIC ENZYMES

In some cases of IBS, the antibiotics mentioned in Chapter 6 that are a core feature of the Cedars-Sinai protocol for IBS may not work. Usually the reason is that the bacteria have developed a resistance to these drugs. In this case, my colleagues and I may have such patients supplement with pancreatic enzymes. Pancreatic enzymes taken with meals can help to digest and break down foods before they pass too far through the gastrointestinal tract, thus starving the bacteria. Typically, patients taking pancreatic enzyme supplements report a

30 to 40 percent improvement in their symptoms over time. This approach is unlikely to eradicate bacterial overgrowth but can reduce it.

ACUPUNCTURE

Acupuncture can be very useful for helping IBS patients cope with many of their symptoms. Both the National Institutes of Health (NIH) and the World Health Organization (WHO), for example, have cited acupuncture as an appropriate treatment for treating symptoms such as abdominal pain, constipation, diarrhea, and muscle cramping.

Acupuncture has also been shown to reduce stress and stress-related problems, such as anxiety, menstrual cramps, and premenstrual syndrome, which can exacerbate the pain and frequency of IBS symptoms.

Acupuncture involves the use of needles inserted in specific points along the body, which run along pathways known as meridians. According to acupuncture theory, the meridians are the pathways through which run a subtle form of vital energy known as *qi* (pronounced "chee"). The purpose of acupuncture is to regulate the flow of *qi* so that it remains balanced, stable, and unblocked, instead of stagnant, excessive, or deficient. The end result, acupuncturists claim, is improved regulation of all of the body's physical processes, increased energy, and improved mental and emotional states. Depending on the needs of the patient, acupuncture treatments can be as short as fifteen minutes and as long as an hour or more, with sessions typically lasting for thirty minutes, with the acupuncture needles remaining in place for most of that time.

Although modern science has now validated acupuncture's ability to provide significant pain relief and to help reduce symptoms of other disease conditions, the scientific explanation remains unknown. Western scientists and physicians who have studied acupuncture theorize that it works by affecting the nervous system, stimulating the release of endorphins, chemicals produced by the body to block pain signals in the brain and spinal cord, and to heighten feelings of well-being and pleasure. Research has also shown that acupuncture produces positive changes in the conduction of electrical signals in the brain, and increases blood flow to the thalamus, a part of the brain that helps regulate and control the relaying of sensory impulses, including pain. Acupuncture has also been shown to regulate the release of neurotransmitters such as norepinephrine and serotonin.

In 2000, researchers presented evidence that acupuncture improved quality-of-life scores and gastrointestinal symptoms among IBS patients, compared with relaxation therapy. In a randomized controlled study involving twenty-seven IBS patients, participants received either acupuncture or relaxation treatments three times a week for two weeks. Both groups reported statistically significant improvements in their abdominal pain at the end of the two weeks, as well as overall improvements in their quality of life. However, after an additional four weeks of follow-up observations, the improvements only persisted among the patients who had received acupuncture. In addition, a statistically significant reduction in stress perception was reported by the acupuncture group, but not by the control group, throughout the study. Based on these results, the researchers who conducted the study concluded that acupuncture is an effective form of treatment for the pain and stress symptoms of IBS, and that its benefits are superior to standard relaxation treatments.

I do not prescribe acupuncture, but based on the scientific evidence I agree that acupuncture may improve IBS symptoms in some cases. If you should choose to receive acupuncture treatments for your IBS, here are some guidelines that you should follow:

- Be sure that the practitioner you choose is properly licensed and credentialed to practice in your state of residence. (Some states allow acupuncturists to work under their own license. Others require that acupuncturists work under the supervision of a licensed physician [MD or DO].)

- Make sure that the practitioner uses only single-use, sterile, disposable needles to prevent the rare but real possibility of infection or the transmission of diseases such as hepatitis.

- Avoid acupuncture if you suffer from an uncontrolled bleeding disorder or are taking anticoagulant medications, such as coumadin, because acupuncture needles have the potential, although rare, to draw blood.

- Be sure to tell your acupuncturist if you are pregnant, as the stim-

ulation of acupuncture points, especially on the stomach, can trigger contractions of the uterus, possibly provoking premature labor
or miscarriage.

- Inform your acupuncturist if you have diabetes, and especially if you
  have diabetic neuropathy. In such cases, acupuncture treatments
  on the arms and legs should be conducted with extreme caution.

LESS-EFFECTIVE TREATMENTS

To conclude this chapter, I wish to briefly mention a few of the more
popular health choices people often make to treat IBS that have little
to no actual value. These include antiflatulent drugs, antidiarrhea
medications, antispasmodic medications, and colonics and enemas.

Antiflatulent Drugs

A number of popular drugs are marketed to reduce gas. Since gas is
often associated with IBS, IBS patients may be tempted to try these
agents. Such products basically break bubbles, but do not get rid of the
gas, so any relief they do provide will be fleeting.

Antidiarrhea Medications

These drugs, including the popular product Imodium, can stop diarrhea symptoms at least temporarily, but they do nothing to address the
root problem of IBS. Using antidiarrhea medications to relieve diarrhea associated with IBS is akin to using morphine to relieve the pain
caused by IBS; neither of these approaches works to resolve IBS. As
a result, I cannot recommend such medications, except perhaps in
extreme situations where diarrhea would otherwise be too uncom-
fortable and/or embarrassing.

Antispasmodic Medications

This class of drugs can be considered attractive to IBS patients who
suffer pain from muscle spasms and cramping. However, like the
drugs mentioned above, the relief they offer is little more than a

Beware of False Hopes: Drugs That Have Little Effect on IBS

In recent years, a variety of drugs have become popular for treating the symptoms of IBS. In most cases, these agents have little or no proven benefit in IBS. One class of such drugs includes the antispasmodics, such as Donnatal and Bentyl. Such drugs are used to relieve the pain and cramping associated with IBS. However, they provide little or no benefit for IBS.

Fiber products are also sometimes prescribed for IBS patients with symptoms of chronic constipation. While getting enough fiber in your diet is certainly an important step to health, a recent meta-analysis of all clinical studies conducted on IBS found that fiber had no major benefit for treating the constipation associated with IBS, and some fiber formulations can even contribute to increased gas and bloating.

IBS patients are also sometimes advised to try products to control flatulence, such as Gas-X. Such products are advertised as being able to reduce gas and hence distension. But all that these products really do is break the gas bubbles. So, instead of the gas being eliminated, the bubbles break and the gas collects in larger pockets. In other words, the quantity of gas itself remains the same.

"Band-Aid" approach for treating IBS, as they are incapable of resolving the underlying cause.

Colonic Therapy and Enemas

Many IBS patients opt to receive colonic therapy or give themselves enemas in an effort to cleanse their lower bowel. Colonic therapy is administered by a trained colon therapist and involves the application of filtered water into the entire length of the colon via a speculum inserted into the rectum. Properly administered, colon therapy can help dislodge fecal matter from the colon, along with fecal microorganisms, including bacteria. Enemas, by contrast, are only able to cleanse the lower, sigmoid colon.

While they can purge the colon of almost all fecal material, thus dramatically reducing the bacterial load in the gut, colonics do not cure IBS and, moreover, are usually not enough to resolve the underlying bacterial overgrowth. There are two reasons for this. First, colonics are incapable of reaching the small intestine, where the offending bacteria live. Secondly, even though colonic therapy can significantly reduce bacteria in the colon, bacteria repopulate very quickly. Some strains are capable of doubling in volume every twenty to thirty minutes, and overall, bacteria can repopulate within one or two days, causing symptoms to return to the same level of severity as before the colonic. Often, patients wind up having repeated colonic sessions without making any true long-term progress in terms of addressing the cause of their IBS symptoms. Enemas are even less effective in this regard.

In addition, colonics are not without risk. I know of cases where patients had to be admitted to the hospital because of rectal bleeding caused by the speculum, either because the patients' rectums were punctured or because they sustained a tear on the rectal surface. If the therapist fails to sterilize the equipment before and after each session, there is also the possibility that patients could contract infectious diseases, including AIDS and hepatitis B or C. For all of these reasons, I do not recommend colonics or enemas.

CONCLUSION

The therapies outlined in this chapter, in many cases, result in a decrease of IBS symptoms, and, in the case of the elemental diet (Vivonex), might even help to resolve bacterial overgrowth altogether. Overall, with the exception of the elemental diet, most of these treatments cannot do more than mask the symptoms. To most effectively address and resolve the bacterial overgrowth that causes IBS, the full Cedars-Sinai protocol for IBS is required.

Now that you understand which alternative therapeutic methods have some degree of value, and which do not, let's examine the relationship between IBS and other conditions, such as fibromyalgia. The link between such diseases is the subject of Chapter 8.

Fibromyalgia and Other Associated Conditions:
The IBS Connection

Many people with IBS also suffer from other health problems, such as fibromyalgia. The reverse is also true. Many people with fibromyalgia suffer from IBS. The link between these two conditions is well established but poorly understood. This chapter sheds light on how IBS and fibromyalgia are connected, and also examines how IBS may play a role in other associated conditions, such as interstitial cystitis and various gynecological problems, as well as fatigue and a lack of mental clarity or "brain fog."

FIBROMYALGIA

Fibromyalgia is a condition characterized by many symptoms. Its primary characteristic is widespread muscle pain caused by the tightening and thickening of the myofascia, the tissues that hold muscles together.

Fibromyalgia is a very complex diagnosis, with no known cause. Compounding the problem is the disparity of opinions within the medical community. If a patient is experiencing muscle aches and pains, the diagnosis they receive can depend upon the doctor's specialty. An internist may tell the patient there is nothing wrong, after medical testing fails to find indications of rheumatological conditions such as rheumatoid arthritis or lupus. Thus, people with fibromyalgia are in a similar situation to IBS patients who are told that their symptoms are "all in their head." In both IBS and fibromyalgia, the patients know that the symptoms they are experiencing are real, but they are given no medical validation, leaving them frustrated and at a loss as to what they can do to help themselves.

On the other hand, if that same patient were to see a rheumatologist, who is oriented to look for fibromyalgia, the symptoms would be tested according to the diagnostic criteria for fibromyalgia. Within this criteria are eighteen so-called tender points in the muscle areas on the body. If eleven or more of these points are tender or painful when the physician presses on them, and if the tenderness continues for at least three months, the patient is said to have fibromyalgia. However, because the cause of fibromyalgia is not known, treating it remains difficult, especially so because of the variance of views about fibromyalgia within the medical community. Some physicians consider it to be due to an overactive immune system, while other physicians maintain it doesn't actually exist. The views run from one extreme to the other.

Overall, just as IBS is a "hot potato" condition in the minds of many gastroenterologists because of how difficult it can be to diagnose and treat, fibromyalgia is a similar "hot potato" for many rheumatologists. Currently, there is no standard treatment for fibromyalgia. The scope of treatments employed by physicians is enormous, ranging from a component of cough syrup to fluconazole (a treatment for systemic yeast infection [candidiasis]), to treatments for Lyme disease. Consequently, most fibromyalgia patients find themselves in a very difficult situation, and yet are determined to find a treatment that can actually help them.

There is a tremendous overlap between IBS and fibromyalgia. Not all IBS patients present with fibromyalgia symptoms, but nearly all fibromyalgia patients have IBS. As a result, there has been a growing amount of interest among researchers to examine whether or not fibromyalgia is linked to IBS. A lot of very good work in this area has been conducted by Dr. Lin Chang at the University of California, at Los Angeles (UCLA).

Given the possible link between IBS and fibromyalgia, my colleagues and I decided to explore whether bacterial overgrowth might be a factor in fibromyalgia, as fibromyalgia appears to have a role in IBS.

In our first study, breath tests were administered to fibromyalgia patients. A higher percentage of them tested positive for elevated levels of bacterial overgrowth compared with control groups. Moreover, subjects with fibromyalgia were noted to suffer from many of the gastrointestinal complaints that are typical of IBS.

But the exciting findings did not occur until we conducted our second study. In that study, which we published in the *Annals of Rheumatology*, we found that fibromyalgia patients had bacterial overgrowth more often than IBS sufferers. Furthermore, fibromyalgia patients had hydrogen levels during breath testing that were the highest we had ever seen; levels significantly higher than non-fibromyalgia IBS patients and, of course, healthy control patients. My colleagues and I were struck by these findings because they show that there *is* a link between bacterial overgrowth and fibromyalgia.

Let's examine how bacterial overgrowth, especially overgrowth of bacteria that produce elevated hydrogen levels, might contribute to fibromyalgia pain.

The initial assumption is that greater hydrogen levels imply that there are more bacteria in the small intestine, which would lead to a greater production of bacterial toxins (endotoxins). These endotoxins enter the bloodstream through the small intestine. We know, from many studies in the scientific literature, that these endotoxins in the bloodstream can enter and affect the liver; there, they are detoxified. However, endotoxin levels can exceed the liver's detoxifying capacity, leading to toxemia, a condition in which toxic substances are spread throughout the body through the bloodstream. This means that bacterial overgrowth beyond a certain threshold produces a corresponding degree of toxemia. We also know that if the degree of toxemia reaches a certain threshold, it can cause pain. Endotoxins, in particular, are well known to cause pain. In studies of rats, for example, it has been shown that when an endotoxin is injected into the skin of rats, they will develop pain not only in the area of the body that is injected, but will also experience pain over their entire bodies. This is the model of pain that can be extrapolated from the research my colleagues and I have conducted that links bacterial overgrowth to fibromyalgia. We believe that the levels of endotoxins in fibromyalgia patients might just exceed the liver's detoxifying capacity and spill over into the bloodstream to cause systemic hyperalgesia, a condition characterized by a heightened sensitivity to pain that closely matches the characteristics of fibromyalgia. Therefore, conducting further research to see if reducing bacterial overgrowth in fibromyalgia patients will also reduce their pain symptoms makes good sense. This is to some degree supported by the fact that our research found a correlation between body pain severity and the level of hydrogen on breath tests.

Though we have not yet conducted a large-scale definitive double-blind study to determine whether the Cedars-Sinai protocol for treating IBS will achieve similar results for fibromyalgia patients, early indications are that it might. In a small, randomized double-blind study that my colleagues and I presented at the American College of Rheumatology meeting in Boston in 1999, we showed that fibromyalgia patients who received the antibiotic drug neomycin, and whose breath tests became normal as a result, also experienced relief from their fibromyalgia symptoms, as evidenced by a significant improvement in their tender point count.

An example of this is the case of a sixty-two-year-old woman who had been given a diagnosis of fibromyalgia ten years before first being seen at the Cedars-Sinai GI Motility Program. She recognized the contribution of her bowel symptoms to her overall condition and after reading our work sought consultation with us. Her breath test showed extremely high hydrogen levels; at the same time, she had fourteen out of eigthteen tender points positive on her physical exam. She then received a course of the antibiotic neomycin. By the time the treatment was completed, her bowel symptoms had resolved, as had her body pain. Using our strategy of prevention, she has remained relatively symptom-free for the last three years.

Based on the results of patients, such as the one mentioned above, who experienced a recovery from their IBS symptoms as well as significant improvements in their fibromyalgia, I am comfortable saying that bacteria overgrowth is a factor physicians ought to consider in cases such as this.

INTERSTITIAL CYSTITIS

Interstitial cystitis, also known as irritable bladder, is a disease characterized by inflammation and irritation of the bladder. Symptoms of interstitial cystitis include frequent urination and dysuria (painful or difficult urination).

Like fibromyalgia, interstitial cystitis has no known cause and is another "hot potato" disease, meaning that many urologists and nephrologists (physicians who specialize in the treatment of kidney disease) are often unable to treat it with consistently reliable results. The use of cytoscopy (in which a cytoscope is placed inside the bladder for diagnostic purposes) sometimes reveals a slightly elevated immune reaction within the bladder lining.

Many patients with IBS are also diagnosed with interstitial cystitis, so there is a degree of overlap between the two conditions. In addition, both conditions are less understood, in terms of their pathophysiology, than fibromyalgia.

We do not yet know whether there is a direct relationship between bacterial overgrowth and interstitial cystitis. But there is one interesting area of research that suggests a potential link. European researchers have shown that the cleansing waves of the small intestine are synchronized with the body's need to urinate. In one study that monitored the cleansing waves of the small intestine for twenty-four hours, the researchers found that 80 to 90 percent of all trips to the bathroom in order to urinate were preceded by cleansing waves of the gut. This finding suggested that the physiological mechanisms that activate the small intestine's cleansing waves may also activate bladder function.

Thus, it is possible that dysfunction of the cleansing-wave mechanisms is in some way linked to bladder dysfunction. If future research shows a correlation between these types of dysfunction, then interstitial cystitis may also be due to the gut movement disturbances seen in IBS that cause bacterial overgrowth. If researchers discover that deficiencies within the cleansing-wave mechanisms cause or contribute to dysfunctions of the bladder, this could explain the overlap between IBS and interstitial cystitis.

GYNECOLOGICAL PROBLEMS

One of the difficulties associated with IBS is that it presents in so many different ways. Abdominal pain is a manifestation of IBS, but pain is a nondescript symptom of many problems in the abdominal and pelvic cavity. Gynecological problems, such as pelvic pain, are a good example of this. Many women with pelvic pain syndromes, for example, experience relief from their symptoms following a healthy bowel movement.

Pelvic pain is a frequent reason for women to seek medical attention from their gynecologist. With up to one in six women suffering from IBS, gynecologists also see many women who have IBS as well as their presenting complaint. Since IBS is very common as are many gynecologic conditions such as endometriosis, this raises a question: Is the pain causing women to visit the gynecologist representing a gynecological problem or might it actually be IBS?

This is a very important question that deserves serious contemplation by patient and gynecologist alike to avoid leading women with IBS symptoms to believe that they have gynecological problems instead.

Mislabeling the patient can result in unwarranted surgical procedures. It's not uncommon for women with IBS to be referred to a gynecologist for symptoms that are mistakenly assumed to be gynecological in origin; for example, endometriosis, ovarian cysts, pelvic inflammatory disease, and various other gynecological conditions cause pain. As a result, invasive gynecological procedures might be performed that fail to address the patient's problem because the real culprit is IBS.

A diagnosis of endometriosis is the best example of this. It is well understood that if endometriosis involves the bowel or rectum, it can result in disturbances of bowel function. In addition, endometriosis can cause pelvic pain. Yet both of these symptoms—disturbed bowel function and pelvic pain—can also be caused by IBS. That being the case, physicians who treat endometriosis-like pain should first ask themselves if it is endometriosis or IBS that is causing the symptoms. The answer may determine whether cauterization or laparoscopic surgery should be performed.

The issue of unnecessary gynecological surgeries due to an underappreciation of the contribution of IBS to pelvic symptoms points to the need for further research in order to understand the overlap that exists between symptoms that are truly gynecological and gynecological-like symptoms that are actually due to IBS. In the meantime, the potential similarities between gynecological and

IBS symptoms is something that women and their physicians need to understand.

One way to encourage the consideration of IBS is to take a bowel symptom history. If the pelvic pain is associated with alterations in bowel function such as diarrhea or constipation (or both), this points to an intestinal cause of symptoms. Moreover, if the pain precedes and is relieved by bowel movements, IBS is again more likely to be the diagnosis. Since both IBS and endometriosis are so common, it is very likely there will be patients with both conditions. This situation is even more complex since the physician must identify which diagnosis is most relevant to the patient's concerns. Is the endometriosis asymptomatic (without symptoms)?

As an aside, I would also like to point out that unnecessary gynecological surgical interventions are not the only type of surgeries that can occur because of undiagnosed IBS. It is not uncommon for IBS patients to undergo other types of unnecessary surgeries, such as having their appendix or gallbladder removed. IBS can present with episodes of increased severity ("attacks of IBS") during which time abdominal pain may be severe, mimicking a more ominous condition such as appendicitis or gallstones.

Birth control pills and menstruation are two other situations of a gynecological nature that can affect IBS and, in turn, be affected by it. Many women with IBS experience fluctuations in their symptoms based on their menstrual cycle. For example, some women with constipation-predominant IBS report that their symptoms improve during their periods or during their premenstrual cycle. In other cases, women report that their symptoms worsen during these times, while still other women experience no change in their symptoms.

This is similar to Crohn's disease (inflammation of the gastrointestinal tract), where one-third of all women with this condition experience a worsening of their symptoms during pregnancy, while another third experience improvements, and the final third find that their symptoms remain the same.

Currently, we do not fully understand why IBS symptoms can be affected for better or worse during or near menstruation, and there is no way to predict if and how such fluctuations will occur. More research is needed to address these questions.

The use of birth control pills can also cause fluctuations in IBS symptoms. Birth control pills influence a woman's hormone levels, which may explain why many women who use birth control pills report changes in their IBS symptoms. Although the medical literature shows that levels of the hormone progesterone can affect the motor function of the gastrointestinal tract—creating a positive effect for some women and a negative effect for others—there is not enough research to explain how and why fluctuations in hormone levels, including those caused by birth control pills, can often cause fluctuations in IBS symptoms as well. In the meantime, we do know that even when hormonal fluctuations improve IBS symptoms, they do not make the symptoms go away.

FATIGUE, "BRAIN FOG," AND HYPOGLYCEMIA

A significant percentage of IBS patients also experience regular bouts of fatigue, in some cases diagnosed as chronic fatigue syndrome (CFS). CFS is an extremely difficult diagnosis to make with any degree of accuracy because fatigue is a common symptom of many conditions. The inability to be certain that one has excluded all possible diseases makes it difficult to study chronic fatigue patients.

Researchers have to decide what to include as criteria for their research protocols. Should they conduct all diagnostic tests related to all of the disease conditions that cause fatigue? In addition, researchers and physicians must also address the problems associated with determining the cause of each patient's fatigue. For example, it is not unusual for a patient who is experiencing fatigue to be told by his or her doctor that there is no discernible cause for the problem. Three years later, additional tests might reveal that he or she has abnormally low thyroid function or is anemic due to vitamin B_{12} deficiency, whereas neither of these causative factors was detectable when the patient was initially tested.

Because cases of fatigue are difficult to diagnose and understand, I cannot say with certainty that there is a direct link between IBS and CFS. However, as mentioned, many IBS patients do complain of being tired and lacking energy. The vast majority of patients that I've treated for IBS, who also complained of fatigue, report that their fatigue significantly improved after they were treated for bacterial overgrowth, using the Cedars-Sinai protocol. Therefore, bacterial overgrowth is something that might be considered when no other factors are found to explain a patient's ongoing fatigue symptoms in the circumstance of fatigue's association with IBS.

Another symptom that is quite common among IBS patients is impaired memory and cognitive function that can best be described as a type of "brain fog." Many of my IBS patients describe this symptom as a feeling of mentally "not being all there." The experience fluctuates to a great degree. Some days, usually when their IBS symptoms aren't as bad, the patients feel fine mentally, but on other days, they feel like they are mentally dragging themselves around. They lack mental focus and feel lethargic. In some cases, they also experience a slight degree of hesitancy with words and have trouble expressing themselves.

In terms of their mental clarity, many IBS patients find that mid to late afternoon is the time when their mental abilities are most noticeably out of focus. Typically, it is during this period of the day when they also feel the most fatigue, often to the point where they feel a need for a nap. One potential explanation for this is hypoglycemia (low blood sugar). Research conducted by my colleagues and me showed that nearly all IBS patients experience some degree of hypoglycemia after a carbohydrate challenge (taking in more carbs than usual to check for a reaction). This is especially pronounced among IBS patients for whom breath testing shows elevated levels of hydrogen in the small intestine. In addition, the degree of patient's hypoglycemia is directly proportional to the degree of bacterial overgrowth that is indicated by breath tests. Although we do not completely understand the reasons for this lack of mental clarity and to what degree it is caused by or associated with the toxemia that results from bacterial overgrowth, my colleagues and I routinely see an improvement of these symptoms in our patients following treatment of the bacterial overgrowth itself. At this time, these reports are purely anecdotal, but this is an area that my colleagues and I are continuing to study.

There is a medical corollary that supports our patients' reported improvements of their mental function following treatment with the Cedars-Sinai protocol for IBS. It is found among patients suffering with liver disease who, as a result, develop encephalopathy, a term used to describe any type of brain dysfunction including mental confusion.

In such cases, the encephalopathy appears associated with the fact that the liver is no longer able to detoxify bacterial toxins that are being produced in the gut and entering the liver. In a healthy person, such toxins are filtered out and eliminated by the liver. But when liver function starts to fail, the liver is unable to do its job; the toxins then travel through the bloodstream to affect other parts of the body, and affect brain function, causing mental confusion.

One of the treatments for encephalopathy due to liver diseases such as cirrhosis involves one or more courses of antibiotics. This approach has been used since the 1960s. When patients with liver disease who are also experiencing mental confusion and fatigue are given an antibiotic such as neomycin, they typically recover their mental alertness and become better oriented in terms of their overall brain function. Usually, their fatigue will also begin to be reversed.

Based on these well-documented mental improvements among liver disease patients who are treated with antibiotics, it is reasonable to speculate that the "brain fog" that many IBS patients experience is being caused by the extreme amount of bacterial overgrowth in the small intestine, which is overwhelming the liver's ability to detoxify. We don't know for certain whether that is the cause of mental dysfunction among so many IBS patients, but what we do know, based on our patients' own anecdotal reports, is that the experience of "brain fog" usually resolves once the bacterial overgrowth is properly addressed.

This is something for IBS patients to be aware of, because all too often, when they mention their experience of "brain fog" to their doctors, the doctors can be dismissive of them and not take their experiences seriously.

I hope, having read the above, that IBS patients with these symptoms will have a better understanding of what might be causing them, as well as now knowing how they might resolve them.

CONCLUSION

The point of this chapter is to emphasize how the symptoms of IBS can masquerade as other symptoms and/or exacerbate them. This is an important aspect of IBS that patients and physicians alike need to consider more carefully. There is a lot more to IBS than its effects on bowel function; it can cause a variety of other symptoms that are often mis-diagnosed as other conditions. As this chapter makes clear, patients with IBS often have difficulties with a lack of mental clarity and alertness, as well as fatigue and muscle and gynecological pain.

In addition, IBS seems to play a role in fibromyalgia, and can often be concomitantly diagnosed with interstitial cystitis, endometriosis, and other gynecological conditions. Knowing the contribution of IBS to the symptoms will undoubtedly prevent unnecessary surgical procedures on IBS patients. The more that physicians come to understand the role that the bacterial overgrowth associated with IBS can cause symptoms (both inside and outside the gut), the more apt they will be to rule out IBS before proceeding to another diagnosis that could lead to unhelpful surgeries. In the meantime, it is my hope that people with IBS will be empowered by the information this chapter contains to raise these issues with their physicians so that they can be spared "all in your head" diagnostic labels that will only delay their finding the relief they are searching for.

CHAPTER 9

Good Questions Deserve Good Answers:
The IBS Forum

In this chapter, I answer the questions that I am most frequently asked by my patients with IBS. The questions stem from their personal concerns and experiences. Based on my discussions with IBS patients around the nation, these concerns and questions are shared by most people with IBS. It is my hope that my answers will be helpful to the many people with IBS who have not been able to find the answers to their problem. In addition, my answers will give validation to patients who often had their concerns and symptoms dismissed as psychological and stress-based.

My IBS is worse when I'm stressed, but even when I am relaxed it's still there. What can I do about this?

The reason I am beginning this chapter with this question is because many people—physicians and patients alike—are convinced that stress exacerbates the symptoms of IBS. One statement from IBS patients triggers the "all in your head" button with the physician: the declaration that "my IBS is worse when I am stressed." The physician then needs to ask the more important question, "But, do you still have symptoms even when you are not stressed?" I cannot deny that stress—any kind of stress—can affect bowel habits, as we mentioned in earlier chapters. For example, a very serious exam, a problem at work, difficult times in your home life, and even a happy event, such as getting married or receiving a promotion, can make anyone's bowels behave differently, perhaps making underlying IBS symptoms worse.

115

This is not unusual, since we also know that stress can affect normal gastrointestinal function—for example, causing diarrhea due to so-called "butterflies" in the stomach. Those effects on the gut were mentioned in Chapter 3 in relationship to cortisol-releasing factor (CRF), a hormone that is produced in the brain in response to stress. As we previously discussed, elevated CRF levels cause the colon to contract excessively. In addition, the stomach will empty more slowly, but most important, CRF also inhibits the cleansing waves of the gut. So under stressful circumstances, the colon will be more active and the cleansing waves will slow down or stop.

Therefore, it is possible that, number one, stress can exaggerate bacterial overgrowth, and number two, it can worsen the diarrhea symptoms that many IBS patients already have. But, again, I must emphasize that stress is not believed to cause IBS, so when the stressful situation resolves, the patient's symptoms may improve but do not go away. The patient still suffers every day. I have many patients who tell me that they'll go to the most relaxing place they know for a couple of weeks on a vacation and yet they still suffer from their IBS symptoms.

So, although alleviating stress will not all by itself resolve IBS problems—as this book makes clear—it still makes good sense to learn how to deal with stress more successfully so that your symptoms can become more manageable. There are many ways to cope with stress, but to describe them in detail is well beyond the scope of this book. Here are some simple guidelines that can help you get started.

• **Practice relaxation exercises.** By regularly practicing relaxation exercises, you will become better able to release stored tension and therefore be less apt to be negatively affected by stress. There are many types of relaxation exercises, as well as many useful books on this subject. Educate yourself about this subject, find the exercise or exercises that work best for you, and make them a part of your daily routine.

• **Breathe.** When we are under stress, typically our breathing patterns become shallow. In many cases, we may even unconsciously start to hold our breath. One of the most effective ways of countering stress is to consciously take deep relaxing breaths as soon as you start to notice yourself becoming stressed. Doing this for a few minutes at a time throughout the day can dramatically improve your stress-coping abilities. In addition, you will be aiding your overall health by increasing your intake of oxygen.

• **Meditate or pray.** Numerous studies have shown the positive health benefits that regular times of meditation and prayer can provide. In the 1970s, Herbert Benson, MD, of Harvard Medical School, published studies showing that meditating as little as ten to twenty minutes each day triggered what he termed "the relaxation response," a physiological release of tension accompanied by less stressful brain-wave activity. There are many methods of meditation. One of the simplest and most effective is to sit comfortably with your eyes closed and gently focus on your breathing. As an additional aid, you can mentally affirm, "I am relaxed and at peace," each time you inhale.

• **Examine your beliefs and attitudes.** Research shows that stress is often caused not because of the events we experience in life, but by the way we subjectively interpret them. Studies also indicate that people who perceive external events as a personal affront are far more likely to suffer from chronic stress. Such people tend to take everything that happens to them personally, when, in fact, many times that is not the case at all. So, if you are feeling stressed or upset by situations in your life, examine your beliefs about them. Is the situation you find yourself in really as bad as you think it is? Many times, the answer is no. Recognizing that can be a powerful way of letting go of upsets, resulting in greater feelings of peace and equanimity.

• **Develop your sense of humor.** The late Johnny Carson once told his television audience, "If you don't have a sense of humor, you better beg, borrow, or steal one, because sometimes it's the only thing that will get you through life." Scientific research confirms his point. People who make a habit of looking for the humorous side of life tend to be happier and therefore less likely to suffer from stress as badly as people who are more pessimistic. Moreover, the laughter that often results from seeing humor in daily life events has actually been shown to provide health benefits, including improved immune function and the release of stored tension.

• **Make time for yourself and your hobbies.** All work and no play will not only make you dull, it can actually make you sick, according to research in the field of mind/body medicine. Make it a priority to spend at least some part of each week doing activities or hobbies you enjoy. Not only will you be happier, you will also be less stressed.

• **Exercise.** Regular exercise is another powerful way of releasing stress and, of course, provides many other health benefits as well. One of the easiest and yet most effective forms of exercise is to take a walk each day.

None of these methods address the bacterial overgrowth that is at the heart of most cases of IBS. Nonetheless, by making them a regular part of your life, you will find yourself becoming much better able to deal with stress, helping to prevent stress from exacerbating your IBS symptoms. In addition, you will also improve your overall health.

My doctor doesn't believe that bacterial overgrowth causes IBS. He's pretty smart, so why should I doubt him?

I am now asked this question much less frequently than before, since numerous investigators are publishing studies that confirm our findings. Thus gastroenterologists are now recognizing the role that bacterial overgrowth plays in IBS. Nevertheless, there are still many physicians who are unfamiliar with this emerging research link between bacterial overgrowth and IBS. In some cases, they dismiss the thought altogether without taking the time to study the evidence.

Having read this book and examined the evidence for yourself, I hope you will realize that there is help that truly addresses your IBS problems. Moreover, it is also important to understand that physicians are inundated with medical information and have a hard time sifting through so many areas of research to draw their own conclusions. This makes them susceptible to the influence of IBS traditionalists.

I am not trying to "push" a theory, but rather to accelerate people's knowledge of a concept with scientific evidence. New concepts take years to be adopted by internists and gastroenterologists. As such, some physicians continue to say things like, "Well, I don't know anything about bacterial overgrowth's being a factor in IBS, so therefore it must not be true."

We should not be so quick to blame physicians for this lack of knowledge but perhaps assist them by giving them opportunities to take interest in the latest information in this area. There are many theories for many conditions, not only IBS, and sorting through all of these theories can be confusing for physicians, as well as for their patients. Many physicians simply do not have time to synthesize the evidence, given their busy schedules.

Though my colleagues and I initially developed the Cedars-Sinai protocol for IBS based on the findings of just a few scientific papers we had published recounting our initial studies, our ultimate goal was to prove that bacterial overgrowth causes the vast majority of IBS cases in double-blind studies, and to confirm our findings to justify the initial study conclusions. More important, other physicians and researchers are now reproducing our findings with their own studies and clinical trials. You can mention such studies to your physician (see the References section).

Compounding the problem about how to most effectively treat IBS is the fact that many physicians, with the best of intentions, look to experts within the medical field to guide them in what is correct and what is not. Unfortunately, sometimes these experts also are unaware of the latest medical research or still express their doubts. This happened when bacterial overgrowth was first proposed as a causative factor for IBS at medical conferences. When certain leading expert gastroenterologists were asked what they thought about it, they made comments like, "I don't think it's real. I think we really need more data. It hasn't convinced me yet, so I'm not treating it that way." Such comments initially delayed the acceptance of the bacterial overgrowth theory of IBS. As physicians, educators, and leading scientists, my colleagues and I have to use our influence to further the medical knowledge based on critical understanding of the scientific data itself, even when it contradicts long-held theories and beliefs.

Finally, as a patient, the criteria you should use in evaluating whether or not your physician is helping you with your health problems is to ask yourself if the treatment protocols he or she recommends are providing you with the relief you are looking for. If, after a reasonable period of time, they are not, then you may need to seek other help or options.

I think I have IBS. How do I get a breath test in my area?

The best way to locate a physician in your area who uses breath testing is to contact QuinTron Instrument Company, the manufacturer of the machines I recommend. They can be reached at:

    QuinTron Instrument Company
    3712 West Pierce Street
    Milwaukee, WI 53215.
    Phone: 800–542–4448 • www.quintron-usa.com.

Two Notes of Caution About Breath Tests

First, be aware that there are some breath testing kits available in which the breath samples are collected in the physician's office and are then mailed to a remote location or lab for analysis. In our experience, the breath samples do not travel well and can lead to some inaccuracies. In-office testing is preferable. The second note of caution relates to how some doctors are conducting breath testing. While the normal test is three hours long, some offices are cutting corners. In fact, I have heard that some doctors take only one breath sample. Apart from the determination of the presence or absence of methane, this does not give enough information.

The normal test involves a baseline breath sample, after which you should be given a sugar syrup (preferably lactulose, although some centers are still using glucose) followed by breath samples every 15–30 minutes for at least 90 minutes but preferably for 180 minutes (3 hours). If this is not happening, then there is reason to be concerned about the quality of your breath test.

Upon contacting them, you will receive an entire list of every center in the whole country that does breath testing or that has at least acquired one of their devices. Preferably, look for a center or physician with a QuinTron Model SC machine, since this model tests for both methane and hydrogen.

Since bacteria seem to be involved in IBS, can I pass IBS on to my family members?

My patients ask me this question very often. When we think of bacteria, we think of it as being contagious in some way, and that it can be contracted by casual or even more intimate contact. The short answer is no. However, if we consider that the IBS sequence (and likely bacterial overgrowth) can be precipitated by food poisoning, we can transmit bacteria that cause food poisoning to somebody else. In fact, that's how food poisoning is transmitted. Improper hand washing and improper food preparation by restaurants and other agents that handle food, such as grocery stores and so forth, create opportunities for passing on pathogenic organisms such as bacteria from one person to another. However, in terms of bacterial overgrowth in IBS, once the food poisoning has done its damage, the resulting bacterial overgrowth itself is not contagious. You can't give it to somebody else. You can't spread IBS from one person to another. That being said, there are people who believe that it runs in families, which brings us to our next question.

Is there a genetic predisposition for IBS?

Currently, the Mayo Clinic is conducting research on genetics as it relates to IBS. The problem with answering this question with any certainty has to do with answering such questions as to whether family members have IBS because of a genetic predisposition or because they all grew up together and were exposed to the same factors, for example got food poisoning with the same pathogens. This is a big issue that's going to be difficult to resolve. I believe it will be very difficult to prove that IBS is genetic because you can't eliminate other factors shared by families, such as meals.

If bacterial overgrowth is a possible explanation for IBS, why isn't IBS rampant in Third-World countries?

This is an excellent question. For example, if *Campylobacter* causes IBS because of a bad case of traveler's diarrhea that leads to bacterial overgrowth, why, since *Campylobacter* is more common in the Third World, isn't IBS occurring in near-epidemic numbers in these countries, compared with the United States and other Western nations? I suspect the answer is that in many Third-World countries, by the age of five everybody has had exposure to *Campylobacter* and/or other pathogens. Children, however, tend to have less severe reactions to such pathogens when they initially are exposed to them, compared with the severe reactions adults can have.

In addition, once children are exposed to such pathogens, they often develop a tolerance to them that minimizes the reactions they might have to future exposures, compared with people who are not exposed to such pathogens until they are adults.

As an example of this—and there have been scientific studies that confirm this—compare the reactions of an adult from the United States and an adult living in India to *Campylobacter* after eating at a restaurant in India. The person from India will most likely experience only a mild case of food poisoning with only one or two days of diarrhea. The person from the United States, on the other hand, will most likely experience a prolonged bout of bloody diarrhea and might end up in the hospital. The difference is that the person from India was probably already exposed to *Campylobacter* as a child, and therefore has developed a tolerance to it. This is akin to the chicken pox. If you develop chicken pox as a child, you might endure discomfort, but for the most part it is not a serious health problem. But if you don't develop chicken pox until you are an adult, the illness is much more intense and, in some cases, life threatening. The same thing is true for the mumps. Mumps among children is not a big deal, since there usually are no lasting consequences. But when adults get the mumps, it can manifest as a much more serious and violent illness, and, among men, it can cause infertility.

Hepatitis A is another good example of what I am talking about. The majority of people who live in Third-World countries have been exposed to hepatitis A when they were children. At most, they might have developed a little bit of jaundice, but in many cases, they didn't even develop that, and they soon got over the disease. Almost every case of a child who gets hepatitis A will resolve without serious consequences. In adults, however, initial exposure to hepatitis A leads to a far more serious condition. Adult-onset hepatitis A can, in some cases, result in fulminant hepatic failure, and may even require a liver transplant.

Therefore, my colleagues and I think that the reason IBS is not more prevalent in Third-World countries (compared with industrialized nations) is because the pathogens that set the stage for IBS to occur cause much more mild immune reactions in children than they do in adults, and, in general, the vast majority of people in such countries are exposed to such pathogens at an early age, helping their immune systems to develop a certain level of immunity to the pathogens as they get older.

Does having IBS increase my risk for colon cancer?

This is an especially important question when people talk about bacterial overgrowth in relationship to IBS. People often ask me, "What will happen if I don't treat my IBS or the bacterial overgrowth? What if I don't want to take an antibiotic? Is something going to happen to me?"

As far as we currently understand IBS, it is a benign condition in terms of progressing to any kind of cancer. In the 1970s, there was some data suggesting that when methane was present during breath testing in humans, or in the colon of humans, there was an increased risk for colon cancer. However, no researchers said for certain that this was due to the methane gas or to the methane-producing organisms. Subsequent studies refuted that possibility and, as far as I know, the issue has never been looked at again.

What I tell my patients is that we don't really know that there is a link between the two diseases, nor do we know if leaving IBS untreated can cause any other type of damage over time. It's really an issue of morbidity rather than mortality. People suffer from IBS, but it does not kill them. However, young productive people with IBS have a compromised quality of life, both socially and at work. So choosing to be treated or not really depends on what sort of quality of life a person wants.

What about other potential links between IBS and inflammatory gastrointestinal conditions such as Crohn's disease and colitis?

When I was first seeing patients with inflammatory bowel disease during my time as a Fellow at Cedars-Sinai, I noticed that many patients with Crohn's disease would say, "You know, I had a lot of nagging bowel symptoms for ten years, but people scoped me and they did barium studies, yet they didn't see anything. Instead, they called my condition IBS. For ten years they've said I had IBS and then, all of a sudden, I started bleeding, and when they scoped me again, they said I have Crohn's disease. Why didn't they detect this ten years ago? How could they have missed it?"

The answer to that is that they didn't miss it. Instead, what happened was that this patient was in what could be called a "prodromal," or initial, phase of Crohn's disease. Unfortunately, we don't really know why there is such a long latent period before Crohn's disease fully manifests. Ulcerative colitis, in comparison, does not have a prodromal phase per se.

According to a study that my colleagues and I conducted, the average prodromal phase for Crohn's disease is approximately seven years, while for ulcerative colitis it is less than a year. As a result, when ulcerative colitis strikes, usually when you go to your doctor he or she is able to diagnose it right away. Crohn's disease is much more difficult to detect in its early stages when, for all intents and purposes, it can present with symptoms very much like those of IBS before it ultimately develops into detectable Crohn's disease.

This is an important point for physicians and patients to remember when it comes to labeling someone with IBS. It's not uncommon, once the label is made, for the patients' gastroenterologists to stop considering other possibilities as their patients continue to experience IBS symptoms. For example, it's understood that a certain proportion of the population will develop colon cancer over time. If a physician is treating an IBS patient who has dealt with IBS for a significant period of time, perhaps fifteen or twenty years, and the patients keeps returning for follow-up checkups and treatments, eventually it behooves the physician, as the patient nears the age of fifty, to remember to also screen for the possibility of colon cancer. This is something that can become overlooked if the physician relies only on the patients' medical charts, which list their symptoms as IBS. Doctors still need to remember that if their patients' IBS symptoms change even slightly that it could be an indication of something else developing, such as Crohn's disease or colon cancer. When you have a very common disease such as IBS, you've got to be mindful that a second condition could develop alongside of it over time.

However, I want to stress that just because a person has IBS, there is no way to say for certain whether he or she *will* go on to develop another, concomitant condition, nor has any direct link been established between IBS and other gastrointestinal conditions. However, if you have IBS and you notice a change in your symptoms, be sure to alert your doctor about this immediately.

My doctor wants to scope me. Do I really need this?

Even prior to our understanding of the bacterial theory of IBS, there were, and continue to be, guidelines on the type of workup physicians should conduct for an IBS patient. The first step was blood tests to check for anemia, a sedimentation rate test to check for any evidence of elevated immune-system activity—or, in other words, inflammation in the body—and then basic chemistry panels to check for kidney failure or sodium or potassium imbalances in the body. Abnormal blood tests, blood in the stool or weight loss are often referred to in the IBS investigative workup as "red flags"—in other words, circumstances in which the physician needs to be more concerned and consider further testing.

The other test that is often recommended is a flexible sigmoidoscopy, which is the use of a short scope inserted up into the colon and doesn't require sedation. The purpose of this test is to be sure that there isn't any inflammation in the colon, or other signs of ulcerative colitis. The decision to conduct a flexible sigmoidoscopy is really a very arbitrary one and, in most cases, is not really necessary.

Contrary to some patients' understanding, for example, physicians very often miss detecting Crohn's disease with a flexible sigmoidoscopy since, in order to do so, it is necessary to look all the way through the colon into the small bowel, where the sigmoidoscope does not reach. It addition, sigmoidoscopies often miss colon cancer that develops on the right side of the colon. In fact, it misses so many different colon disorders that the role of flexible sigmoidoscopy in general is now being questioned. Therefore, the primary question to consider is when *should* physicians scope a patient? One of the things that I look for in this regard is whether or not a patient's IBS symptoms fluctuate. It doesn't matter if their IBS symptoms are constipation predominant or diarrhea predominant, or in between; I am looking for changes in their symptom patterns that might indicate the development of some other type of health problem. This is a gray area, because no IBS patient has identical symptoms from day to day. One thing that is absolutely characteristic of IBS is the number of bowel movements that IBS patients have from day to day. One day, they may have two bowel movements; the next day they might have only one; the day after that, they might not have any; and on day four, they might have three or four. Such fluctuations aren't really abnormal when it comes to IBS. But if a patient comes to me and says, "I'm having ten diarrheal bowel movements a day, every single day," then that's a worrisome symptom to me and merits a colonoscopy, because IBS, generally speaking, doesn't behave that way. In IBS there is always some degree of fluctuation in the number of the patient's daily bowel movements.

Just as important, if a patient suddenly starts to experience constipation to the point where he or she is having only one very hard bowel movement a week and this never changes, then that's of concern to me, too, and I'm more apt to investigate further. The other scenario where I'm apt to investigate further, and to consider looking for the possibility of celiac disease with a scope that biopsies the small bowel from above, and maybe doing a colonoscopy, as well, is when I treat the patient's bacterial overgrowth and it comes back immediately. Or when I do the breath test and the patient doesn't have bacterial overgrowth at all, and therefore bacterial overgrowth is not the explanation for his or her symptoms. Overall, however, I think performing the breath test first to determine whether or not bacterial overgrowth is present actually increases your likelihood of detecting other possible conditions.

Summing up, if you notice a change in your IBS symptoms, getting scoped might be advisable, but rather than suggesting a uniform rule of thumb, I prefer to make that decision on a case-by-case basis, depending on each patient's current symptoms status.

Why do I feel worse when I have milk products, but even when I completely eliminate them from my diet my IBS symptoms still persist?

There has been some research from Europe suggesting that part of IBS development may be due to lactose intolerance. Among my own patients, if I were to quantitate lactose intolerance symptoms, approximately 80 percent of them either avoid milk and dairy products altogether or recognize that milk and dairy foods are an issue in terms of creating more bloating for them. Yet, even when they eliminate milk and dairy products from their diets, they still have IBS. The only difference is that when they drink milk, their bloating symptoms become worse.

Part of the reason for this has to do with the fact that most bacteria rely on sugar as their main ingredient in terms of nourishment. If bacteria could have only one food, sugar would be the one thing they would want. When a person drinks one cup of milk, the amount of lactose it contains requires almost the entire length of the small intestine to absorb it. Humans are all relatively deficient in the enzyme lactase necessary to assimilate lactose, and as we age, our lactose intolerance becomes even more pronounced because our stores of lactase are reduced over time. Therefore, if you have an overgrowth of bacteria and you eat sugar that reaches the farthest parts of the small bowel, it will further feed the bacterial overgrowth. As the bacteria feed on this sugar, they ferment it, creating gas. My colleagues and I have shown this in a study in which, when we conducted breath tests with lactose, the breath test profile looked identical to the same patient getting a lactulose breath test to look for bacterial overgrowth, meaning that what you're seeing on the lactose breath test using milk sugar is really bacterial overgrowth. We then compared this to the actual lactose tolerance test, which is the gold standard for determining whether or not a person can assimilate lactose. Only three out of twenty IBS patients had true lactose intolerance based on the tolerance test. This points out the fact that using the lactose breath test to screen for lactose intolerance isn't actually accurate because what the test is likely demonstrating is bacterial overgrowth in most cases.

To return to the question at hand, eliminating milk and other dairy products will not, in and of itself, resolve the problem of IBS. In many instances, however, it can help to reduce the symptoms of bloating associated with IBS, because doing so will reduce the amount of sugar the bacteria have available to feed on. A better solution, of course, would be to address the bacterial overgrowth directly. See Chapter 6 for dietary suggestions that may help.

Will a gluten-free diet help my symptoms?

A gluten-free diet is used to treat celiac disease, which has symptom similarities to IBS. To a somewhat lesser degree, this diet is similar to the popular Atkins Diet in the sense that, in both diets, the person is reducing carbohydrates (sugars). In the case of a gluten-free diet, you are switching your carbohydrates more to potato starches and to rice, and therefore to more simple carbohydrates. The complex carbohydrates are the ones that come from grain cereals, and that's where gluten, which is believed to be the protein that causes celiac disease, comes from. Some people often feel that they might have celiac disease, even though all their tests for it came back negative, because they do feel somewhat better on a gluten-free diet. This makes sense because, when you eliminate gluten-containing foods, you are also eliminating complex carbohydrates, and carbohydrates, like sugar, are what bacteria thrive upon. If you starve bacteria of carbohydrates, they cannot sustain their large numbers, so the degree of bacterial overgrowth actually drops, which, we believe, is what explains why IBS symptoms, including bloating, are less pronounced. Again, though, while a gluten-free diet may provide benefit for IBS patients, it rarely is enough for eliminating the bacterial overgrowth, which should be the primary aim of any IBS treatment program.

To some extent we have confirmed this concept in principle. In a study we published recently, we were able to completely eradicate bacterial overgrowth and facilitate a dramatic improvement in IBS using the nutritional product Vivonex (see Chapter 6 for full details). Vivonex is an elemental diet, which means the food that it contains is already completely predigested. Therefore, when a person consumes this product, the food is absorbed so readily into the blood that it does not travel much beyond the first two feet of small intestine (the absorbing area of the gut of which there are fifteen feet). In the case of bacterial overgrowth where, in most cases, the bacteria are further into the small intestine than two feet, taking this type of food starves them and they cannot continue to exist. The overall ability to get rid of bacterial overgrowth with this type of diet for two weeks is nearly 90 percent. The problem is that this diet is very difficult to tolerate even for brief periods of time.

Why is my IBS worse with menstruation?

This is another one of the questions that I am asked frequently. Unfortunately, this is also a phenomenon that we have little understanding about. The truth is that we really don't know why women have alterations in their IBS symptoms based on their menstrual cycle. Some women say that during menstruation, their symptoms—whether they are constipation or diarrhea predominant—improve, while others say their symptoms become worse. Why this is so remains to be determined. We do know, though, that progesterone, which is one of the hormones involved in the menstrual cycle, has motility effects. That's been proven scientifically.

Progesterone is also one of the hormones that are responsible for nausea and vomiting during the first trimester of pregnancy because it causes movement disturbances of the stomach. So we know progesterone plays a role here as well, in terms of IBS and menstruation, but how exactly it does so remains unknown. But researchers are looking into it.

Is there anything I can do during menstruation to minimize my IBS symptoms?

Once we've gotten rid of bacterial overgrowth, we actually don't see as much fluctuation during the menstrual cycle. Therefore, the treatment approach that we've been discussing throughout this book, which targets and eliminates bacterial overgrowth, is the best way of dealing with this issue.

Why do my IBS symptoms, such as bloating, become worse when I'm on an airplane? Because of this, I'm afraid to fly. What should I do if I have an attack on the plane?

I've been told by many of my IBS patients that they are afraid to fly because they are worried that they are going to have a flare-up of their symptoms on the plane. For example, if you have a sudden onset of diarrhea, going to the bathroom on the plane is not that easy because sometimes IBS patients need to spend extra time in the bathroom, to the consternation of their fellow passengers.

In addition, sometimes the diarrhea, when it occurs, can be very foul and therefore disturbing to other passengers, creating an embarrassing situation for the person with IBS, as well as a lot of anxiety. Many IBS patients also often experience an attack of diarrhea within an hour or so after eating. On top of all of these factors that people with IBS have to take into account when they fly, almost all drinks that are served on airplanes contain carbonation, which can exacerbate the bloating and distension of IBS sufferers even more. In my experience, I would say the majority of IBS sufferers just avoid eating on planes for this reason, either because they don't feel that they can handle the meal, or because they worry that something else might happen symptomatically that they won't be able to control. Sometimes, too, there's such a dramatic urgency with IBS that you can't afford to be standing in the back of a plane in a line waiting to use the bathroom. You have to get to it now. All of these factors compound an IBS patient's problems when he or she flies.

As for bloating, because the air pressure inside the plane is not the same as the air pressure as on the ground—the air pressure inside the plane is slightly lower than normal sea level (it's set at typical pressure of an altitude of about 10,000 feet)—IBS patients have a tendency to distend more because the stomach is at a higher level of pressure relative to the outside environment, making bloating and abdominal distension more pronounced once the plane is in the air.

Is there anything I can do to minimize the consequences of flying?

Unfortunately, there isn't any treatment available for bloating besides the treatment of the bacterial overgrowth that I've outlined in this book. Therefore, if a patient is not willing to treat their bacterial overgrowth, then they really don't have any other type of effective treatment option, other than to avoid eating before and during flight times, something that can be impractical during longer flights. Taking Imodium is common practice for diarrhea-predominant IBS patients. In my experience, once the bacteria overgrowth is properly treated and eliminated, flying is usually no longer an issue and antidiarrhea medications aren't necessary.

Conclusion

In the last ten years a revolution has begun in the study of IBS. This is highlighted by numerous research findings that suggest IBS is not a psychological problem. Patients are tired of hearing that IBS is "all in their head" and that they need to learn to "live with it" because we (physicians) have nothing to offer. IBS patients should not be dismissed and may soon not need to "live with it." In this book, I have highlighted the latest discoveries in IBS that are rational and scientifically proven. Specifically, I discussed the latest developments surrounding the association between IBS and gut bacteria.

There is a distinct relationship between having acute gastroenteritis (food poisoning or travelers' diarrhea) and the development of IBS. A significant percentage of people who get an infectious case of diarrhea will go on to develop IBS, suggesting that in certain cases of IBS, food poisoning is the cause. In this book we discussed the case for food poisoning in precipitating IBS and what to do about it.

More important, this book has summarized the data showing that most IBS patients test positive for bacterial overgrowth. This is a situation whereby bacteria that are commonly found in the large intestine now also inhabit parts of the usually sterile small intestine, leading to the symptoms of IBS. The evidence presented demonstrates how treatment of bacterial overgrowth dramatically improves IBS. We call this technique the Cedars-Sinai protocol for IBS.

The hope is that this book empowers those with IBS to realize there is reason for optimism, reason to stop suffering in silence, reason to stop "living" with IBS, and reason to think about treating IBS again. IBS is a stigmatized condition by the nature of having gas, bloating, and bowel dysfunction: symptoms that fall prey to ridicule. It is time for IBS to be recognized as a legitimate condition that can benefit from new theories and treatment strategies.

Glossary

Acupuncture. An alternative or complementary therapy, originating in ancient China, involving the insertion of thin needles through the skin at certain points on the body to relieve pain and other various symptoms.

Acute. Not long lasting; temporary.

Adrenaline. A hormone produced in the adrenal glands that is released into the bloodstream during times of stress.

Alternative therapy. A nonstandard treatment used in place of conventional medicine.

Alveoli. Air sacs in the lungs.

Amino acids. The building blocks of protein.

Anemia. A red blood cell deficiency.

Aspartame. An artificial sweetener used as a sugar substitute.

Asymptomatic. Without symptoms.

Bacterial overgrowth theory of IBS. A theory in which it is supposed that the various symptoms of IBS are caused by an overgrowth of bacteria (normally relegated to the colon) in the small intestine.

Benign disease. A disease that is not life threatening.

Bowels. *See* Large intestine; Small intestine.

Brain fog. Impaired memory and cognitive function.

Brain-gut access. The link between the brain and the gut.

Calcium channel blocker. A drug that blocks the entry of calcium into cells, thereby causing muscles to relax.

Candidiasis. A systemic yeast infection.

Celiac disease. A gastrointestinal disorder caused by sensitivity to gluten, with symptoms that include diarrhea and maldigestion/malabsorption of nutrients.

Chronic. Long lasting and/or recurrent.

Chronic fatigue syndrome (CFS). A disorder with no known cause, characterized by chronic exhaustion, weakness, and depression.

Colitis. Inflammation of the large intestine.

Colon. *See* Large intestine.

Colonic therapy. The application of filtered water into the entire length of the colon via a speculum inserted into the rectum for cleansing purposes.

Colonoscopy. A procedure in which a colonoscope is placed inside the colon for diagnostic purposes.

Complementary therapy. A nonstandard treatment used alongside conventional medicine.

Constipation-predominant IBS. A classification of irritable bowel syndrome in which the patient experiences mostly constipation.

Control group. In a clinical trial, the subjects who do not receive the treatment being studied and serve as a comparison.

Corn syrup. *See* Fructose.

Cortisol-releasing factor (CRF). A hormone that is produced in the brain in response to stress.

Crohn's disease. A condition of chronic inflammation in the gastrointestinal tract.

Cytoscopy. A procedure in which a cytoscope is placed inside the bladder for diagnostic purposes.

Diagnosis of exclusion. A diagnosis that can be made only after all other possible conditions have been eliminated.

Diarrhea-predominant IBS. A classification of irritable bowel syndrome in which the patient experiences mostly diarrhea.

Distal. Farthest from the point of origin.

Duodenum. The highest part of the upper bowel.

Dysuria. Painful or difficult urination.

Elemental diet. A diet in which only water and a predigested meal-replacement product are consumed for the purpose of eliminating bacterial overgrowth.

Encephalopathy. Any type of brain dysfunction, including mental confusion.

Endocarditis. Infection of the heart valve.

Endometriosis. A condition in which the type of tissue lining the uterus (endometrium) grows outside the uterus.

Endorphins. Chemicals produced by the body to block pain signals in the brain and spinal cord, and are also associated with heightened feelings of well-being and pleasure.

Endoscopy. Direct visualization of the intestines or other internal body structures with cameras.

Endotoxins. Harmful bacterial byproducts.

Enema. The application of filtered water into the sigmoid colon for cleansing purposes.

Enzyme. Protein molecules responsible for stimulating chemical reactions in the body.

Erythrocyte sedimentation rate (ESR) test. Measures the speed at which erythrocytes settle and can help determine if inflammation is present in the body.

Erythrocytes. Mature red blood cells that play a role in transporting oxygen to, and carbon dioxide from, the cells, organs, and tissues.

Fibromyalgia. A condition characterized by widespread muscle pain caused by the tightening and thickening of the myofascia, as well as many other symptoms, including irritable bowel syndrome.

Food poisoning. An acute illness of vomiting and/or diarrhea that occurs after eating toxin-contaminated food or drink.

Fructose. A simple sugar found mostly in fruit.

Gastroenteritis. Inflammation of the stomach and intestines.

Gastroenterologist. A physician who specializes in disease of the gastrointestinal tract.

Gastroesophageal reflux disease (GERD). A digestive disorder in which gastric acid flows from the stomach into the esophagus.

Gastrointestinal tract. The system of organs involved in the process of digestion, including the mouth, esophagus, stomach, small intestine, colon, rectum, and anus.

Glucose. A simple sugar; the main source of energy for the body.

Gluten. A component in wheat.

Gut. *See* Large intestine; Small intestine.

Gut hyperalgesia. Heightened pain sensitivity in the gut.

Gynecologist. A physician who specializes in treating disorders of the female reproductive organs.

Heralding episode. An event that triggers the development of a disorder. Also called heralding event or trigger event.

Heterogeneous condition. A condition that can manifest in seemingly opposite ways.

Hypoglycemia. Low blood sugar.

Ileocecal valve. A valve that prevents matter from flowing back from the large intestine to the small intestine.

Interstitial cystitis. A condition characterized by inflammation and irritation of the bladder. Also known as irritable bladder.

Irritable bladder. *See* Interstitial cystitis.

Irritable bowel syndrome (IBS). A functional disorder of the colon and intestines that is characterized by abdominal pain, bloating, diarrhea and/or constipation, gas, and urgency.

Ischemic colitis. Inflammation of the colon due to decreased blood flow to the colon.

Lactase. The enzyme the body uses to break down and digest lactose (milk sugar) in the small intestine.

Lactose intolerance. The inability to digest lactose.

Lactose. A simple sugar found in milk and other dairy products.

Lactulose. Synthetic sugar.

Large intestine. Part of the gastrointestinal tract; a long, tube-like organ connected to the small intestine at one end and to the anus at the other end.

Lymphocytes. Small white blood cells used by the body to fight infection.

Maltitol. A sweetener made from corn used as a sugar substitute.

Maltose. A sugar obtained from malted grains.

Mannitol. A sugar alcohol used as a sugar substitute.

Meta-analysis. An analysis of data from two or more studies.

Migrating motor complex (MMC). The third phase of small-bowel movement that occurs during periods of not eating.

Myofascia. Tissue that holds muscles together.

Nephrologist. A physician who specializes in diseases of the kidneys.

Neurotransmitter. A brain chemical responsible for communication between nerve cells.

Oligosaccharides. A class of carbohydrate that can contribute to bloating.

Pathogenic bacteria. Bacteria that are capable of causing disease.

Pathologist. A physician who specializes in the diagnosis of disease.

Peptic ulcer. Damage to the stomach lining generally caused by a bacteria known as *H. pylori.* Also called stomach ulcer.

Peristalsis. The wavelike movements of muscles that push solids and liquid through the gastrointestinal tract.

Placebo. A pill that does not contain any actual active ingredients.

Placebo effect. A change that occurs either physiologically or emotionally in a person due to the use of a substance that has no special properties; thought to be invoked by the power of suggestion.

Polyps. Small, abnormal growths sometimes found in the colon and rectum.

Post-infectious IBS. IBS that occurs after an episode of food poisoning or parasitic infection.

Probiotics. So-called good bacteria; often taken in supplemental form.

Prodromal phase. The initial stage of a disease.

Progesterone. A female hormone that can have an effect on the motor function of the gastrointestinal tract.

Rectal hyperalgesia. Heightened pain sensitivity in the rectum.

Rectum. The last section of the large intestine, leading to the anus.

Relaxation response. A physiological release of tension accompanied by less stressful brain-wave activity.

Rheumatologist. A physician who specializes in disorders characterized by inflammation or pain in muscles, joints, or fibrous tissue.

Serotonin. A hormone that controls peristalsis, among its various functions in the body.

Sigmoid colon. The lower part of the colon that connects to the rectum.

Sigmoidoscopy. A procedure in which a sigmoidoscope is placed inside the sigmoid colon for diagnostic purposes.

Small intestine. The section of the gastrointestinal tract between the stomach and the large intestine where most digestion occurs.

Sorbitol. A sugar alcohol used as a sugar substitute.

Stomach ucler. *See* Peptic ulcer.

Strictures. Narrowing of the abdomen.

Substance P. A chemical compound believed to be the chemical that increases hypersensitivity in the gastrointestinal tract and lowers the pain threshold in the rectum.

Sucralose. A no-calorie sweetener made from sugar.

Sucrose. Table sugar.

Systemic hyperalgesia. A condition characterized by a heightened sensitivity to pain.

Tardive dyskinesia. A condition characterized by permanent facial contortion.

Thalamus. A part of the brain that helps regulate and control the relaying of sensory impulses, including pain.

Toxemia. A condition in which endotoxins and other toxic substances are spread throughout the body through the bloodstream.

Traveler's diarrhea. A case of food poisoning during travel, usually resulting in diarrhea that lasts for several days.

Ulcerative colitis. Inflammation of the large intestine, resulting in ulcers in the lining of the colon.

Urologist. A physician who specializes in diseases of the urinary tract.

Vagotomy. A medical procedure that involves the administration of pharmaceutical drugs to prevent function of the vagus nerve, which helps to control motor and sensory function.

Xylose. A simple sugar extracted from wood or straw used as a sugar substitute.

References

Acupuncture. National Institutes of Health. Consensus Statement 1997; 15: 1–34.

Agreus L, Svardsudd K, Nyren O, et al. Irritable bowel syndrome and dyspepsia in the general population: overlap and lack of stability over time. *Gastroenterol* 1995;109:671–80.

Balsari A, Ceccarelli A, Dubini F,et al. The fecal microbial population in the irritable bowel syndrome. *Microbiologica* 1982;5:185–94.

Bardhan KD, Bodemar G, Geldof H, et al. A double-blind, randomized, placebo-controlled dose-ranging study to evaluate the efficacy of alosetron in the treatment of irritable bowel syndrome. *Alim Pharm Ther* 2000;14:23–34.

Bearcroft CP, Perrett D, Farthing MJ. Post-prandial plasma 5-hydroxytryptamine in diarrhoea predominant irritable bowel syndrome: a pilot study. *Gut* 1998;42:42–6.

Betram S, Kurland L, Lydick E, et al. The patient's perspective of irritable bowel syndrome. *J Fam Pract* 2001;50:521–5.

Bohmer CJ, Tuynman HA. The clinical relevance of lactose malabsorption in irritable bowel syndrome. *Eur J Gastroenterol Hepatol* 1996;8:1013–6.

Bommelaer G, Poynard T, Le Pen C, et al. Prevalence of irritable bowel syndrome (IBS) and variability of diagnostic criteria. *Gastroenterol Clin Biol.* 2004; 28:554–61.

Bradette M, Pare P, Douville P, et al. Visceral perception in health and functional dyspepsia. Crossover study of gastric distension with placebo and domperidone. *Dig Dis Sci* 1991;36:52–58.

141

Bradley HK, Wyatt GM, Bayliss CE, et al. Instability in the fecal flora of a patient suffering from food-related irritable bowel syndrome. *J Med Microbiol* 1987;23:29–32.

Bueno L, Fioramonti J. Effects of corticotropin-releasing factor, corticotropin and cortisol on gastrointestinal motility in dogs. *Peptides* 1986;7: 73–77.

Cahill CM, Dray A, Coderre TJ. Priming enhances endotoxin-induced thermal hyperalgesia and mechanical allodynia in rats. *Brain Res* 1998;808: 13–22.

Camilleri M, Mayer EA, Drossman DA, et al. Improvement in pain and bowel function in female irritable bowel patients with alosetron, a 5-HT3 receptor antagonist. *Alim Pharm Ther* 1999;13:1149–59.

Chun A, Desautels S, Slivka A, et al. Visceral algesia in irritable bowel syndrome fibromyalgia, and sphincter of oddi dysfuntion, type III. *Dig Dis Sci* 1999;44:631–636.

DeCross AJ, Marshall BJ. The role of helicobacter pylori in acid-peptic disease. *Am J Med Sci* 1993;306:381–392.

Drossman DA, McKee DC, Sandler RS, et al. Psychosocial factors in the irritable bowel syndrome. A multivariate study of patients and nonpatients with irritable bowel syndrome. *Gastroenterol* 1988;95:701–708.

Drossman DA, Patrick DL, Whitehead WE, et al. Further validation of the IBS-QOL: a disease-specific quality-of-life questionnaire. *Am J Gastroenterol* 2000; 95:999–1007.

Drossman DA, Richter JE, et al., eds. Functional gastrointestinal disorders: diagnosis, pathophysiology and treatment: a multinational consensus. Boston: Little, Brown, 1994.

Drossman DA, Ringel Y, Vogt BA, et al. Alterations of brain activity associated with resolution of emotional distress and pain in a case of severe irritable bowel syndrome. *Gastroenterol* 2003;124:754–761.

Drossman DA, Sandler RS, McKee DL, et al. Bowel patterns among subjects not seeking health care. *Gastroenterol* 1982;83:529–534.

El-Serag HB. Impact of irritable bowel syndrome: prevalence and effect on health-related quality of life. *Rev in Gastroenterol Dis* 2003;3 (Suppl 2):S3–11.

Fass R, Longstreth GF, Pimentel M, Fullerton S, Russak SM, Chiou C-F, Reyes E, Crane P, Eisen G, McCarberg B, Ofman J. Evidence and consensus-based practice guidelines for the diagnosis of irritable bowel syndrome. *Arch Intern Med* 2001;161:2081–88.

Gaby AR. *Altern Med Rev* 2003;8:3.

Gade J, Thorn P. Paraghurt for patient with irritable bowel syndrome. A controlled clinical investigation fromgeneral actice. *Scand J Prim Health Care* 1989;7:23–26.

Galatola G, Grosso M, Barlotta A, et al Diagnosis of bacterial contamination of the small intestine using the 1g [14] xylose breath test in various gastrointestinal diseases. *Minerva Gastroenterol Dietol* 1991;37:169–175.

Gershon MD. Review article: serotonin receptors and transporters—roles in normal and abnormal gastrointestinal motility. *Aliment Pharmacol Ther* 2004;20:3–14.

Goldstein R, Braverman D, Stankiewicz H. Carbohydrate malabsorption and the effects of dietary restriction on symptoms of irritable bowel syndrome and functional bowel complaints. *Israel Med Assoc J* 2000;2:583–587.

Gwee KA. Wee S. Wong ML. Png DJ. The prevalence, symptom characteristics, and impact of irritable bowel syndrome in an Asian urban community. *Am J Gastroenterol* 2004;99:924–931.

Halpert A, Toner BB, Whitehead WE, et al. Cognitive behavioral therapy versus education and desipramine versus placebo for moderate to severe functional bowel disorders. *Gastroenterol* 2003;125:19–31.

Harraf F, Schmulson M, Saba L, et al. Subtypes of constipation predominant irritable bowel syndrome based on rectal perception. *Gut* 1998;43:388–394.

Hungin AP, Whorwell PJ, Tack J, Mearin F. The prevalence, patterns and impact of irritable bowel syndrome: an international survey of 40,000 subjects. *Aliment Pharm Ther.* 2003;17:643–650.

Husebye E, Hellstrom PM, Sundler F, et al. Influence of microbial species on small intestinal myoelectric activity and transit in germ-free rats. *Am J Physiol* 2001;280:G368–80.

Jones MP, Craig R, Olinger E. Small intestinal bacterial overgrowth is associated with irritable bowel syndrome: the cart lands squarely in front of the horse. *Am J Gastroenterol* 2001;96:3204–5.

Kanaan SA, Saade NE, Haddad JJ, et al. Endotoxin-induced local inflammation and hyperalgesia in rats and mice: a new model for inflammatory pain. *Pain* 1996;66:373–379.

Kellow JE, Eckersley GM, Jones M. Enteric and central contributions to intestinal dysmotility in irritable bowel syndrome. *Dig Dis Sci* 1992;37: 168–174.

Kellow JE, Gill RC, Wingate DL. Prolonged ambulant recordings of small bowel motility demonstrate abnormalities in the irritable bowel syndrome. *Gastroenterol* 1990;98:1208–18.

Kellow JE, Phillips SF. Altered bowel motility in irritable bowel syndrome is correlated with symptoms. *Gastroenterol* 1987;92:1885–93.

Kim HJ, Camilleri M, McKinzie S, et al. A randomized controlled trial of probiotic, VSL #3, on gut transit and symptoms in diarrhea-predominant irritable bowel syndrome. *Alim Pharmacol Ther* 2003;17:895–904.

King TS, Elia M, Hunter JO. Abnormal colonic fermentation in irritable bowel syndrome. *Lancet* 1998;352:1187–89.

Koide A, Yamaguchi T, Odaka T, et al. Quantitative analysis of bowel gas using plain abdominal radiograph in patients with irritable bowel syndrome. *Am J Gastroenterol* 2000;95:1735–41.

Kumar D, Wingate DL. The irritable bowel syndrome: a paroxysmal motor disorder. *Lancet* 1985;Nov 2:873–877.

Lea R, Houghton LA, Reilly B, et al. Is abdominal bloating related to physical distension in patients with irritable bowel syndrome (IBS). *Gastroenterol* 2003; 142:A14.

Lea R, Whorwell PJ. Quality of life in irritable bowel syndrome. *Pharmacoeconomics* 2001;19:643–653.

Lemann M, Dederding JP, Flourie B, et al. Abnormal perception of visceral pain in response to gastric distension in chronic idiopathic dyspepsia. The irritable stomach syndrome. Dig Dis Sci 1991;36:1249–54.

Lembo T, Munakata J, Nabiloff B, et al. Sigmoid afferent mechanisms in patients with irritable bowel syndrome. *Dig Dis Sci* 1997;42:1112–20.

Lind CD. Motility disorders in the irritable bowel syndrome. *Gastroenterol Clin North Am* 1991;20:279–295.

Logan AC, Beaulne TM. *Altern Med Rev* 2002;7:410–417.

Lu B, Hu Y, Tenner S. A randomized controlled trial of acupuncture for irritable bowel syndrome. Program of the 65th Annual Scientific Meeting of the American College of Gastroenterology, 2000, New York, NY.

Malinen E, Rinttila T, Kajander K, et al. Analysis of the fecal microbiota of irritable bowel syndrome patients and healthy controls with real-time PCR. *Am J Gastroenterol* 2005;100:373–382.

Manning AP, Thompson WG, Heaton KW, et al. Towards positive diagnosis of the irritable bowel syndrome. *Br J Med* 1978;2:653–654.

Mayer EA, Gebhart GF. Basic and clinical aspects of visceral hyperalgesia. *Gastroenterol* 1994;107:271–293.

McKee DP, Quigley FM. Intestinal motility in irritable bowel syndrome: is IBS a motility disorder? Part 1. Definition of IBS and colonic motility. *Dig Dis Sci* 1993;38:1761–72.

McKee DP, Quigley FM. Intestinal motility in irritable bowel syndrome: is IBS a motility disorder? Part2. Motility of the small bowel, esophagus, stomach, and gall-bladder. *Dig Dis Sci* 1993;38:1773–82.

Mearin F, Cucala M, Azpiroz F, et al. The origin of symptoms on the brain-gut axis in functional dyspepsia. *Gastroenterol* 1991;101:999–1006.

Mertz H, Morgan V, Tanner G, et al,. Regional cerebral activation in irritable bowel syndrome and control subjects with painful and nonpainful rectal distention *Gastroenterol* 2000;118:842–848.

Mertz H, Nabiloff B, Munakata J, et al. Altered rectal perception is a biological marker of patients with the irritable bowel syndrome. *Gastroenterol* 1995; 109:40–52.

Munakata J, Nabiloff B, Harraf F, et al. Repetitive sigmoid stimulation induces rectal hyperalgesia in patients with irritable bowel syndrome. *Gastroenterol* 1997;112:55–63.

Nabiloff BD, Mayer EA. Sensational developments in irritable bowel syndrome. *Gut* 1996;39:770–771.

Neal KR, Barker L, Spiller RC. Prognosis in post-infectious irritable bowel syndrome: a six year follow up study. *Gut* 2002;51:410–413.

Neal KR, Hebden J, Spiller R. Prevalence of gastrointestinal symptoms six months after bacterial gastroenteritis and risk factors for development of the irritable bowel syndrome: postal survey of patients. *BMJ* 71997; 314: 779–782.

O'Mahony L, McCarthy J, Kelly P, et al. Lactobacillus and bifidobacterium in irritable bowel syndrome: symptom responses and relationship to cytokine profiles. *Gastroenterol* 2005;128:541–551.

Patrick DL, Drossman DA, Frederick IO, et al. Quality of life in persons with irritable bowel syndrome: development of and validation of a new measure. *Dig Dis Sci* 1998;43:400–411.

Pimentel M, Chow EJ, Hallegua D, Wallace D, Lin HC. Small intestinal bacterial overgrowth: A possible association with fibromyalgia. *J Musculoskeletal Pain* 2001;9:107–113.

Pimentel M, Chow EJ, Lin HC. Eradication of small intestinal bacterial overgrowth reduces symptoms of irritable bowel syndrome. *Am J Gastro* 2000;95:3503–06.

Pimentel M, Chow EJ, Lin HC. Normalization of lactulose breath testing correlates with symptom improvement in irritable bowel syndrome: A double-blind, randomized, placebo controlled study. *Am J Gastroenterol* 2003;98: 412–419.

Pimentel M, Constantino T, Kong Y, Bajwa M. An elemental diet is highly effective in normalizing the lactulose breath test in patients with bacterial overgrowth. *Dig Dis Sci* 2004;49:73–77.

Pimentel M, EJ Chow, P Hassard, JJ Ofman, S Fullerton and HC Lin. The prevalence of Irritable bowel syndrome in subjects with gastroesophageal reflux disease. *J Clin Gastroenterol* 2002;34:221–224.

Pimentel M, Hallegua D, Wallace D, Chow E, Kong Y, Park S, Lin HC. A link between irritable bowel syndrome and fibromyalgia may be related to findings on lactulose breath testing. *Annals Rheumat Dis* 2004;63: 450–452.

Pimentel M, Kong Y, Park S. Breath testing to evaluate lactose intolerance in IBS correlates with lactulose testing and may not reflect true lactose malabsorption. *Am J Gastroenterol* 2003;98:2700–04.

Pimentel M, Kong Y, Park S. IBS subjects with methane on lactulose breath test have lower post-prandial serotonin levels than hydrogen. *Dig Dis Sci* 2004; 49:84–87.

Pimentel M, Mayer AG, Park S, Chow EJ, Hasan A, Kong Y. Methane production during lactulose breath test is associated with gastrointestinal disease presentation. *Dig Dis Sci* 2003;48:86–92.

Pimentel M, Soffer EE, Chow EJ, Lin HC. Lower frequency of MMC is found in IBS subjects with abnormal breath test suggesting bacterial overgrowth. *Dig Dis Sci* 2002;47:2639–43.

Prior A, Maxton DG, Whorwell PJ. Anorectal manometry in irritable bowel syndrome: differences between diarrhoea and constipation predominant subjects. *Gut* 1990;31:458–462.

Rajagopalan N, Kurian G, John H. Symptom relief with amitriptyline in the irritable bowel syndrome. *J Gastroenterol Hepatol* 1998;13:738–741.

Richter JE, Barish CF, Castell DO. Abnormal sensory perception in patients with esophageal chest pain. *Gastroenterol* 1986;91:845–852.

Ritchie J. Pain from distension of the pelvic colon by inflating a balloon in the irritable colon syndrome. *Gut* 1973;14:125–132.

Robson KM, Kakullavarapu J, Lembo T. Bacterial overgrowth and irritable bowel syndrome: a look at prevalence, symptoms and quality of life. *Am J Gastroenterol* 2003;98:S271.

Saggioro A. Probiotics in the treatment of irritable bowel syndrome. *J Clin Gastroenterol* 2004;38:s104–106. Saggioro A. Erratum. *J Clin Gastroenterol* 2005;39:261.

Shaw AD, Davies GJ. Lactose intolerance: problem in diagnosis and treatment. *J Clin Gastroenterol* 1999;28:208–216.

Silverman DH, Munakata JA, Ennes H, et al. Regional cerebral activity in normal and pathological perception of visceral pain. *Gastroenterol* 1997; 112:64–72.

Simren M, Ringstrom G, Agerforz P, et al. Small intestinal bacterial overgrowth is not of major importance in the irritable bowel syndrome. *Gastroenterol* 2003;124:A163.]

Spiller RC. Postinfectious irritable bowel syndrome. *Gastroenterol* 2003; 124: 1662–71.

Spiller RC, Jenkins D, Thornley JP, et al. Increased rectal mucosal enteroendocrine cells, T-lymphocytes, and increased gut permeability following acute Campylobacter enteritis and in post-dysenteric irritable bowel syndrome. *Gut* 2000;47:804–811.

Steffen R, Sack DA, Riopel L, et al. Therapy of travelers' diarrhea with rifaximin on various continents. *Am J Gastroenterol* 2003;98:1073–78.

Steinhart MJ, Wong PY, Zarr ML. Therapeutic usefulness of amitriptyline in spastic colon syndrome. *Int J Psychiatry Med* 1981;11:45–57.

Stotzer PO, Bjornsson ES, Abrahamsson H. Interdigestive and postprandial motility in small-intestinal bacterial overgrowth. *Scand J Gastroenterol* 1996; 31:875–880.

Szurszewski JH. A migrating electric complex of the canine small intestine. *Am J Physiol* 1969;217:1757–63.

Tabas G, Beaves M, Wang J, et al. Paroxetine to treat irritable bowel syndrome not responding to high-fiber diet: a double-blind, placebo-controlled trial. *Am J Gastroenterol* 2004;99:914–920.

Tache Y. Corticotropin releasing factor receptor antagonists: potential future therapy in gastroenterology? *Gut* 2004;53:919–921.

Thompson DG, Laidlow JM, Wingate DL. Abnormal small-bowel motility demonstrated by radiotelemetry in a patient with irritable colon. *Lancet* 1979;Dec 22:1321–23.

Thompson WG. The functional gastrointestinal bowel disorders. In DA Drossman (ed.) The functional gastrointestinal disorders. Boston, Little, Brown, 1994, pp117–134.

Thompson WG, Heaton KW. Functional bowel disorders in apparently healthy people. *Gastroenterol* 1980;79:283–288.

Tolliver BA, Jackson MS, Jackson KL, et al. Does lactose intolerance really play a role in the irritable bowel syndrome. *J Clin Gastroenterol* 1996;23:15–17.

Vantrappen G, Janssens J, Hellemans J, Ghoos Y. The interdigestive motor complex of normal subjects and patients with bacterial overgrowth of the small intestine. *J Clin Invest* 1977;59:1158–66.

Vasinder GB, Stolk MF, Ke MY, et al. Micturition is associated with phase III of the interdigestive migrating motor complex in man. *Am J Gastroenterol* 2003; 98:66–71.

Viewpoint on Acupuncture. World Health Organization. Geneva, Switzerland; 1979.

Vernia P, Ricciardi MR, Frandina C, et al. Lactose malabsorption and irritable bowel syndrome. Effect of a long term lactose-free diet. *Ital J Gastroenterol* 1995;27:117–121.

Vesa TH, Seppo LM, Marteau PR, et al. Role of irritable bowel syndrome in subjective lactose intolerance. *Am J Clin Nutr* 1998;67:710–715.

Walker K, Dray A, Perkins M. Development of hyperthermia and hyperalgesia following intracerebroventricular administration of endotoxin in the rat: effect of kinin B1 and B2 receptor antagonists. *Immunopharmacology* 1996;33:264–269.

Walsh JW, HAsler WL, Nugent CE, et al. Progesterone and estrogen are potential mediators of gastric slow-wave dysrhythmias in nausea of pregnancy. *Am J Physiol* 1996;270:G506–G514.

Wang SX, Wu WC. Effects of psychological stress on small intestinal motility and bacteria and mucosa in mice. *World J Gastroenterol* 2005; 11:2016–21.

Whitehead WE, Holtkotter B, Enck P, et al. Tolerance for rectosigmoid distension in irritable bowel syndrome. *Gastroenterol* 1990;98:1187–92.

Whitehead WE, Palsson OS. Is rectal pain sensitivity a biological marker for irritable bowel syndrome: Psychological influences on pain perception. *Gastoenterol* 1998;115:1263–71.

Wilson S, Roberts L, Roalfe A, et al. Prevalence of irritable bowel syndrome: a community survey. *Br J Gen Pract.* 2004;54:495–502.

Xiao ZL, Pricolo V, Biancani P et al. Role of progesterone signaling in the regulation of G-protein levels in female chronic constipation. *Gastroenterol* 2005; 128:667–675.

Index